Fragrance

and

Fashion

Published in the United States by
TODTRI Book Publishers
254 West 31st Street
New York, NY 10001-2813
Fax: (212) 695-6984
E-mail: info@todtri.com

Visit us on the web!
www.todtri.com

ISBN 1-57717-205-1

Packaged by De Agostini Rights/meb_hildy

Cover design by White Space Graphic Design

Printed and bound in Korea

Fragrance
and
Fashion

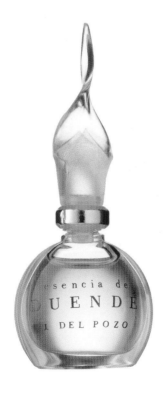

Table of Contents

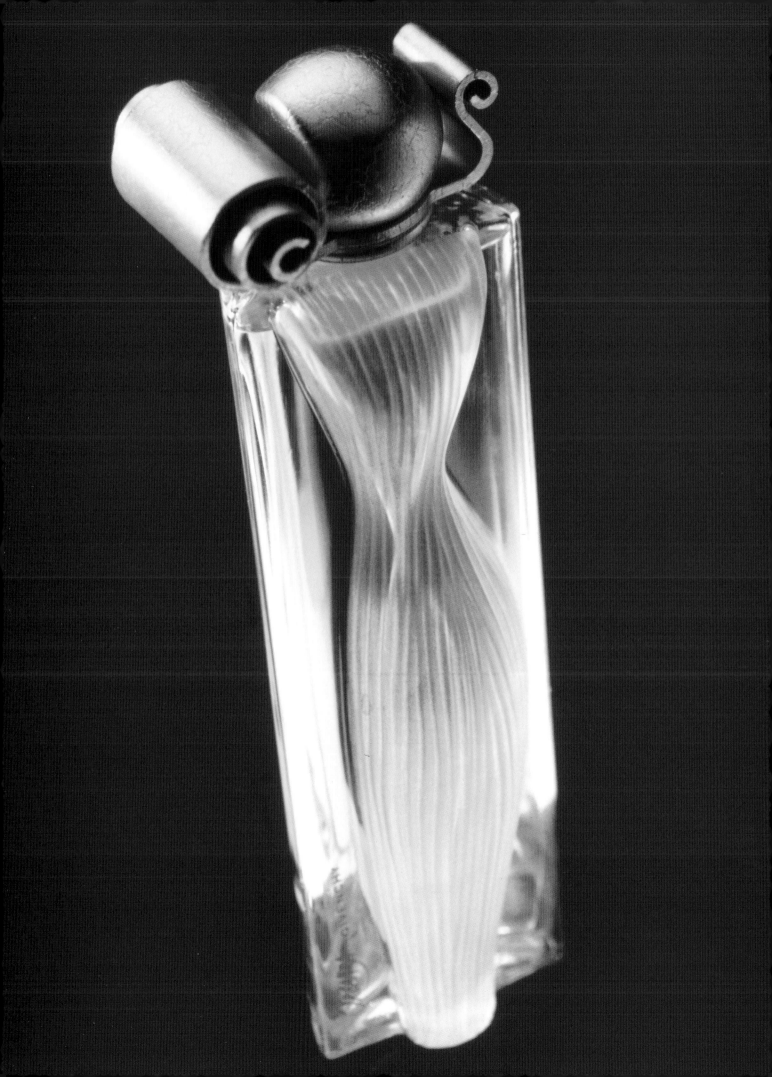

AN INTRODUCTION TO FRAGRANCE AND FASHION

Sometimes controversial, always fascinating – detailed profiles of the major designers, fashion houses and perfumers who create the fragrances worn by millions of men and women. Each study features a history of the perfumer or fashion house, a chronological profile of the genius behind the name, plus influential clients and muses.

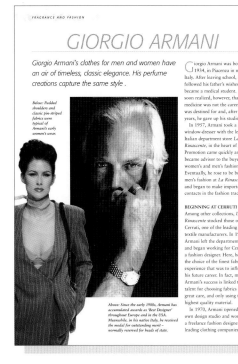

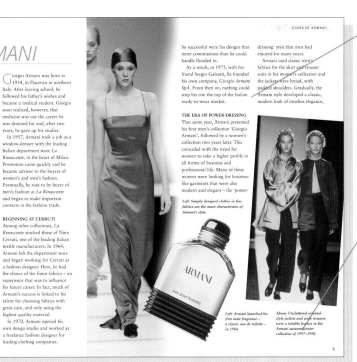

FRAGRANCE & FASHION

Many modern perfumers began their careers as fashion designers or cosmetics gurus – or vice versa. This irresistible combination often sets the scene for an intoxicating tale of glamour and ambition.

SECRET OF SUCCESS

A successful scent can catapult a designer to untold riches and power. Discover the secrets of the men and women whose vision captures the imaginations of millions.

COLLECTION

The beautiful models, clever image campaigns and carefully marketed bottles that define the type of person who might wear a particular perfume.

PROFILE

Chronological profiles of the image-makers and their perfumes: historical background, career development, notable achievements.

GIORGIO ARMANI

Giorgio Armani's clothes for men and women have an air of timeless, classic elegance. His perfume creations capture the same style.

Below: Padded shoulders and classic pin-striped fabrics were typical of Armani's early women's wear.

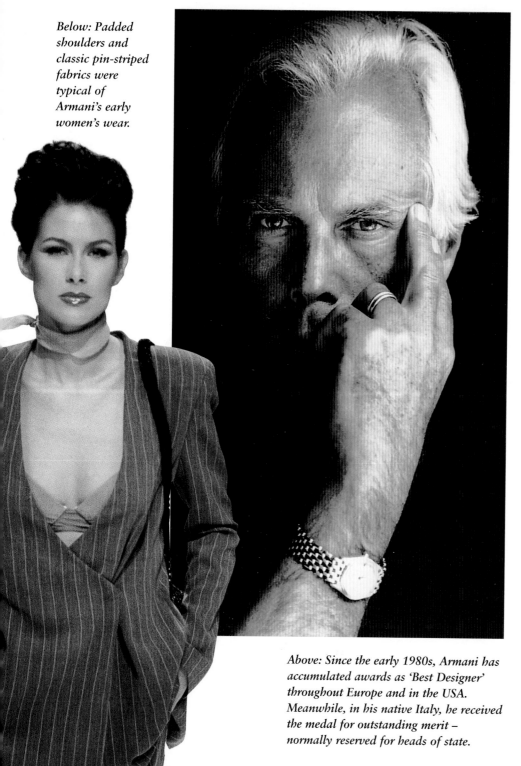

Above: Since the early 1980s, Armani has accumulated awards as 'Best Designer' throughout Europe and in the USA. Meanwhile, in his native Italy, he received the medal for outstanding merit – normally reserved for heads of state.

Giorgio Armani was born in 1934, in Piacenza in northern Italy. After leaving school, he followed his father's wishes and became a medical student. Giorgio soon realized, however, that medicine was not the career he was destined for and, after two years, he gave up his studies.

In 1957, Armani took a job as a window-dresser with the leading Italian department store *La Rinascente,* in the heart of Milan. Promotion came quickly and he became advisor to the buyers of women's and men's fashion. Eventually, he rose to be buyer of men's fashion at *La Rinascente* and began to make important contacts in the fashion trade.

BEGINNING AT CERRUTI

Among other collections, *La Rinascente* stocked those of Nino Cerruti, one of the leading Italian textile manufacturers. In 1964, Armani left the department store and began working for Cerruti as a fashion designer. Here, he had the choice of the finest fabrics – an experience that was to influence his future career. In fact, much of Armani's success is linked to his talent for choosing fabrics with great care, and only using the highest quality material.

In 1970, Armani opened his own design studio and worked as a freelance fashion designer for leading clothing companies.

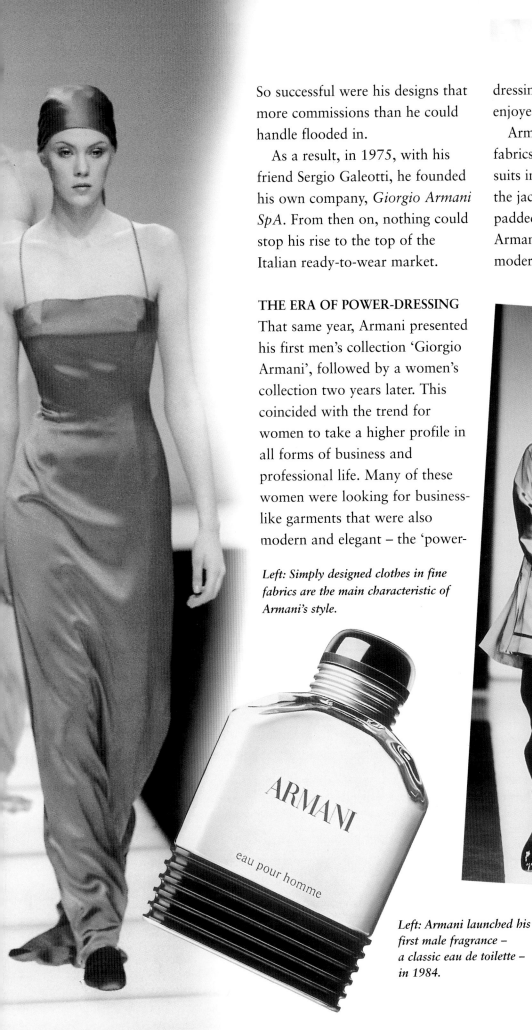

So successful were his designs that more commissions than he could handle flooded in.

As a result, in 1975, with his friend Sergio Galeotti, he founded his own company, *Giorgio Armani SpA*. From then on, nothing could stop his rise to the top of the Italian ready-to-wear market.

THE ERA OF POWER-DRESSING
That same year, Armani presented his first men's collection 'Giorgio Armani', followed by a women's collection two years later. This coincided with the trend for women to take a higher profile in all forms of business and professional life. Many of these women were looking for business-like garments that were also modern and elegant – the 'power-

Left: Simply designed clothes in fine fabrics are the main characteristic of Armani's style.

dressing' style that men had enjoyed for many years.

Armani used classic men's fabrics for the skirt and trouser suits in his women's collection and the jackets were broad, with padded shoulders. Gradually, the Armani style developed a classic, modern look of timeless elegance,

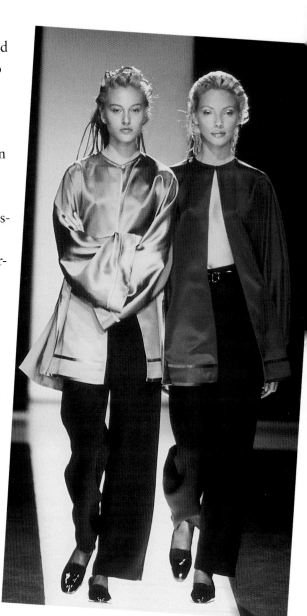

Left: Armani launched his first male fragrance – a classic eau de toilette – in 1984.

Above: Uncluttered oriental-style jackets and wide trousers were a notable feature in the Armani autumn/winter collection of 1997–1998.

Right: In 1982, Giorgio Armani launched his first women's fragrance. Armani has a chypre bouquet with fresh green and cool floral notes.

Below: The men's fragrance Armani eau pour homme, *with its leathery, woody base, was launched in 1984.*

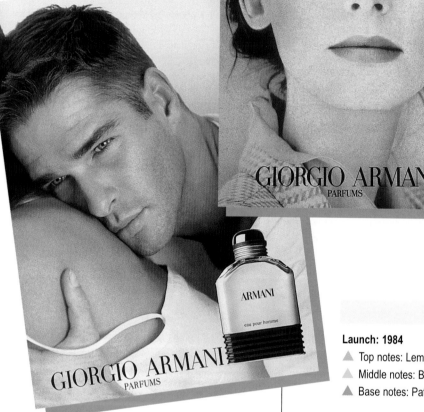

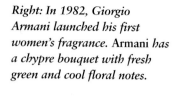

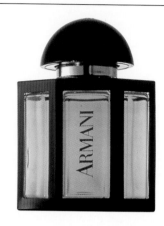

Giorgio Armani
COLLECTION

ARMANI

Launch: 1982
▲ Top notes: Spearmint, Galbanum
▲ Middle notes: Jasmin, Lily-of-the-Valley
▲ Base note: Musk
Style: Summer-like and floral and, at the same time, classic and sporty-elegant. It is the perfect expression of modern Italian style.

ARMANI POUR HOMME

Launch: 1984
▲ Top notes: Lemon, Mandarin, Petitgrain
▲ Middle notes: Bay, Carnation, Jasmin
▲ Base notes: Patchouli, Vetiver, Moss

Style: A fresh and long-lasting fragrance. This classic, cool eau de toilette has a lively freshness, with citrus notes complemented by a slightly floral and woody bouquet.

with its logo: 'Style is more important than fashion.'

As his success grew, Armani also launched accessories and – in line with many other fashion designers – his own perfumes.

PERFUMES TRUE TO STYLE

With his fragrances, Armani remained true to his individual style. In 1982, he marketed his first women's perfume, called *Armani*, a classic floral fragrance with sporty, elegant nuances. Two years later, the men's equivalent appeared.

In 1992, *Giò* was launched – a floral and fruity female fragrance, which bears Armani's signature twofold. He created the design for the bottle, reminiscent in shape of his characteristically broad-shouldered jackets, and he had his nickname, 'Giò', printed on the bottle in his own handwriting.

At the launch, Armani transformed 5,500 square metres of New York's most expensive quarter into an exotic sultan's palace. Supermodels and film stars ensured massive media interest.

His TV advertisements were directed by film-makers David Lynch (*Twin Peaks*) and Martin Scorsese (*Taxi Driver*). Armani knows the power of the media and how to use them for his purposes.

In his private life, Giorgio Armani is said to be a shy workaholic with an iron discipline. He lives alone in a wing of his Milan palace, which is also the headquarters of his worldwide business. His hard work and classic collections are the keys to the success of his empire.

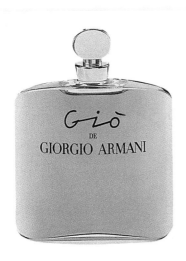

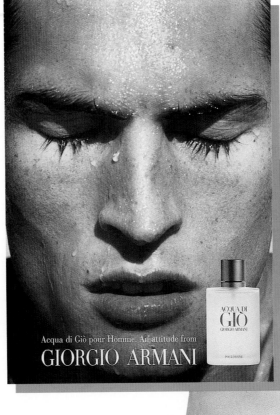

Acqua di Giò pour Homme. An attitude from
GIORGIO ARMANI

Left: Acqua di Giò pour homme *is* evocative of cool green water.

Below: Armani's advertising proclaims that 'A perfume is worthless without the human skin.'

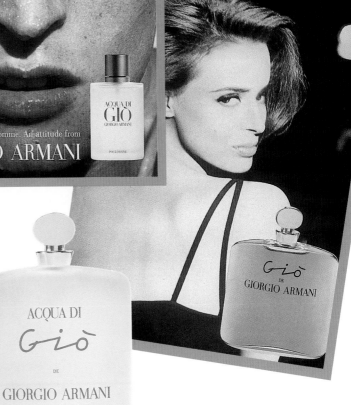

GIÒ

Launch: 1992

▲ Top notes: Bergamot, Mandarin, Peach
▲ Middle notes: Ylang-Ylang, Rose, Tuberose, Carnation, Jasmin, Orris
▲ Base notes: Cedar, Musk, Amber

Style: A classic, floral, fruity perfume with a romantic, warm and intoxicating bouquet.

ACQUA DI GIÒ

Launch: 1995

▲ Top notes: Sweet-salty, Sweet pea
▲ Middle notes: Jasmin, Hyacinth, Freesia, Nutmeg
▲ Base notes: Exotic woods

Style: An aquatic-floral eau de toilette – even its blue and green bottle is reminiscent of cool water.

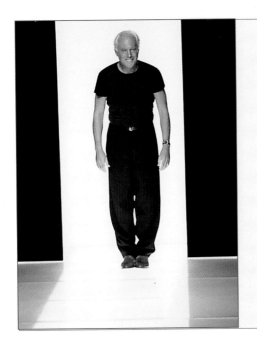

PROFILE

Giorgio Armani

1934 Giorgio Armani born in Piacenza, northern Italy.
1957 Starts work at the department store La Rinascente, Milan.
1964 Designs 'Hitman' collection for Nino Cerutti.
1970 Opens his own design studio.
1975 Founds his own company, Giorgio Armani SpA, in partnership with Sergio Galeotti. Launches first men's collection 'Giorgio Armani'.
1977 Launch of his first women's collection.
1982 US magazine *Time* publishes cover story about Armani.

PERFUME CHRONOLOGY

1982	*Armani* (women)	**1995**	*Acqua di Giò* (women)
1984	*Armani eau pour homme* (men)	**1996**	*Acqua di Giò pour homme* (men)
1992	*Giò* (women)		

11

COCO CHANEL

In the 1920s, Coco Chanel not only revolutionized women's fashion with her easy-to-wear clothes and fabulous costume jewellery, she also produced the world's most famous scent – Chanel Nº 5.

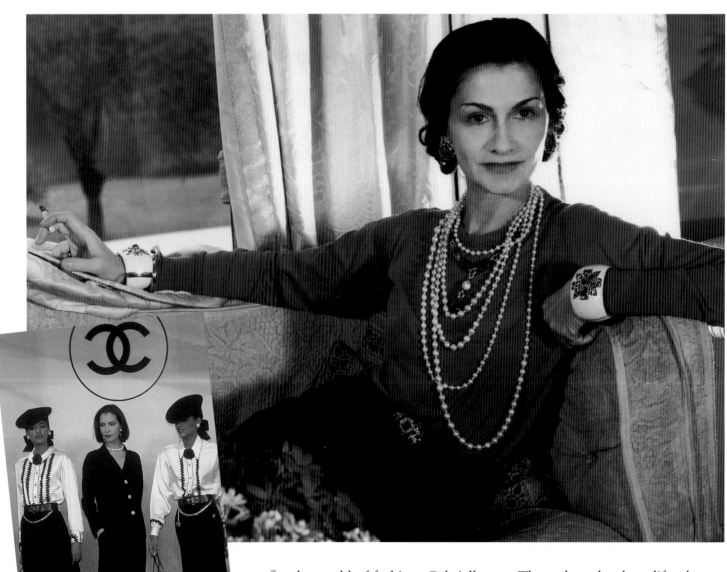

Above: Chanel's elegant look, echoed in these 1990s designs (inset), is timeless. Her logo of entwined Cs is still used by the fashion house.

In the world of fashion, Gabrielle 'Coco' Chanel is almost immortal. She pioneered enduring fashions such as short skirts, the 'little black dress', glittering costume jewellery and, above all, the most celebrated perfume in the world – *Chanel Nº 5*.

Throughout her long life, she was also a source of much speculation due to her 'scandalous' love affairs. She took up with a cavalry officer when she was a cabaret dancer in Vichy, for example. Later, she had an affair with the wealthy Duke of

Westminster, who helped her to set up her first fashion house. Her most controversial love affair was with a young German army officer during the occupation of Paris. This liaison resulted, at the end of World War II, in Chanel facing a charge of collaboration. She managed to emerge relatively

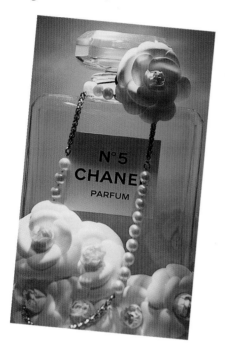

Above: The Chanel Nº 5 *bottle and label is the essence of classic chic.*

unscathed, having pleaded '*l'amour*' as a defence. Chanel concocted many stories about her life – and glossed over many facts – but the truth was sometimes more sensational than the fiction.

FASHION BREAKTHROUGH
After her stint as a cabaret dancer in Vichy, where she became known as 'Coco', Chanel moved to Paris. There, she met Beau Capel – a handsome, wealthy young man who died young and whom she came to regard as the love of her life. Capel helped her to set up a

hat shop at 21 rue Cambon, which quickly became fashionable.

Soon after this she opened a boutique in Deauville, the fashionable seaside resort on the Normandy coast, where she began to produce the loose-fitting, easy-to-wear casual clothes that made her famous.

A NEW AGE OF DESIGN
At the time, Chanel and her designs were daring: she threw away the corset, cut her hair short like a boy's, wore men's trousers and allowed her skin to be tanned by the sun. Her clients loved the simplicity and elegance of her clothes, in marked contrast to the elaborate, restrictive garments of the time. Soon, fashion magazines began to take notice and Chanel's trademark jersey suits, with their long cardigan-style jackets, became all the rage in Paris.

Among her other creations during the 1920s and '30s were the 'little black dress', long ropes of fake pearl costume jewellery, plus bangles and brooches made of paste, diamonds and rubies. For her female garments she chose fabrics such as tweed and gabardine which, until then, had been the preserve of men's tailoring.

A NEW TYPE OF PERFUME
Chanel's greatest stroke of genius was the launch of the world's first 'synthetic' perfume. In 1921, she was approached by Ernest Beaux, a young chemist who, for many years, had studied aldehydes –

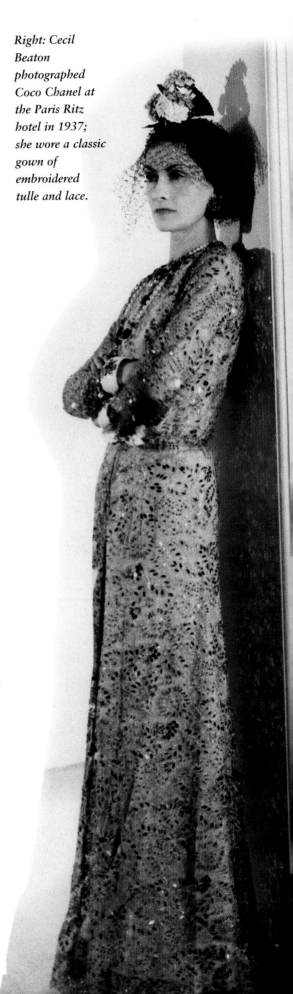

Right: Cecil Beaton photographed Coco Chanel at the Paris Ritz hotel in 1937; she wore a classic gown of embroidered tulle and lace.

Coco Chanel

1883	Gabrielle Chanel born in Saumur, France
1910	Sets up a hat shop in rue Cambon under the label Chanel Mode
1913	Establishes fashion shop in Deauville
1924	The Chanel Perfume Co set up
1926	Introduces 'the little black dress'
1930	Signs contract with Sam Goldwyn to dress stars of United Artists
1954	Makes comeback by opening a new shop in rue Cambon
1971	Coco Chanel dies on 10 January

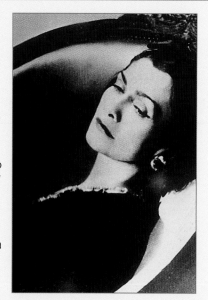

PERFUME CHRONOLOGY

1921	*Chanel Nº 5 and Nº 22*	**1981**	*Antaëus pour homme*
1955	*Pour Monsieur*	**1984**	*Coco*
1970	*Chanel Nº 19*	**1990**	*Égoïste*
1974	*Cristalle*	**1996**	*Allure*

synthetic substances which were able to develop and intensify the natural fragrances of flowers during the distillation process.

Chanel agreed to try some of his samples and Beaux duly put together different fragrances, which he presented to her in numbered bottles. Legend has it that Chanel chose the fifth bottle because five was her lucky number. To continue the superstition, she launched it on 5 May, 1921 – the fifth day of the fifth month of the year.

A DEMOCRATIC PERFUME

Chanel Nº 5 was an immediate success. It remains one of the most celebrated scents in the world and represented a real revolution in the world of perfume. Its lovely freshness made natural essences seem rather old-fashioned and very expensive. Chanel had launched the world's first 'democratic' perfume. Women all over the world loved it and even those of modest means could afford it. Today, almost all the world's perfumers use aldehydes.

Chanel was obliged to close her fashion house during World War II, but she reopened it in the mid-1950s and triumphed again.

THE GRAND TRADITION

Chanel introduced nothing particularly new after the '30s, simply variations on her famous little black dress and woven suits. However, the most elegant women in the world still wear her designs.

Coco Chanel died in 1971, but her successor Karl Lagerfeld carries on her grand tradition.

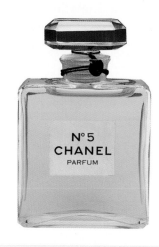

CHANEL Nº 5

Launch: 1921
▲ Top notes: Aldehyde, Bergamot
▲ Middle notes: Lily-of-the-valley, Jasmin
▲ Base notes: Vetiver, Sandalwood
Style: The classic floral perfume, in its elegant bottle, is timeless, sensual and feminine.

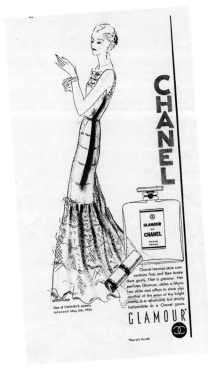

Above: An advertisement for Glamour, *launched in the USA in 1934, sells a sophisticated lifestyle as well as a fragrance.*

CHANEL Nº 19

Launch: 1970

▲ Top notes: Galbanum, Hyacinth, Neroli

▲ Middle notes: Rose, Orris, Jasmin

▲ Base notes: Vetiver, Oakmoss, Leather

Style: With its woody base notes and vibrant green top notes, this subtle and complex fragrance exudes a hint of violet amid its floral elegance.

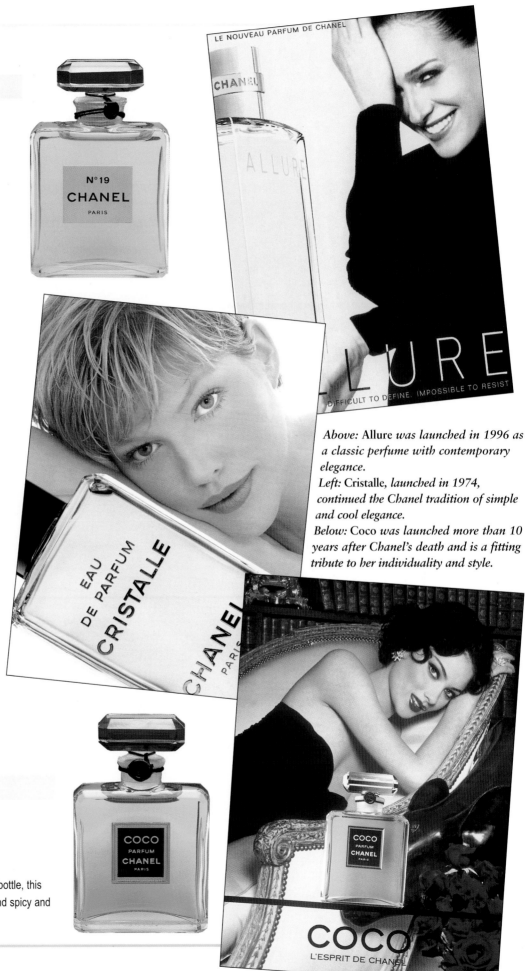

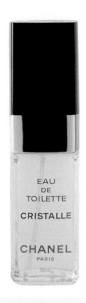

CRISTALLE

Launch: 1974

▲ Top notes: Bergamot, Lemon

▲ Middle notes: Jasmin, Melon, Narcissus, Cyclamen, Lily-of-the-valley, Tangerine

▲ Base notes: Oakmoss, Musk, Civet

Style: Fresh and light, this is a classic chypre perfume with a mossy base.

COCO

Launch: 1984

▲ Top notes: Fruit Notes, Mandarin

▲ Middle notes: Rose, Carnation

▲ Base notes: Olibanum, Amber, Benzoin

Style: Contained in the characteristic Chanel bottle, this modern, long-lasting perfume is both warm and spicy and sweet and floral, with oriental hints.

Above: Allure *was launched in 1996 as a classic perfume with contemporary elegance.*

Left: Cristalle, *launched in 1974, continued the Chanel tradition of simple and cool elegance.*

Below: Coco *was launched more than 10 years after Chanel's death and is a fitting tribute to her individuality and style.*

ESTÉE LAUDER

Estée Lauder's rise from working in a beauty parlour to successful businesswoman was based on determination and innovative ideas. Her perfume, Youth Dew, was the first fragrance that women bought for themselves.

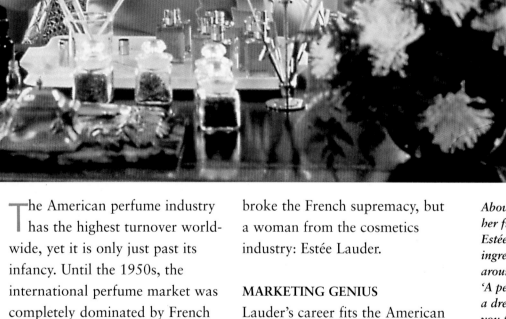

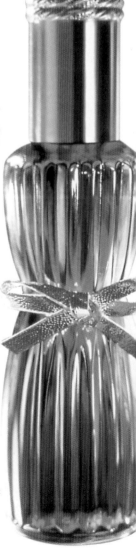

The American perfume industry has the highest turnover world-wide, yet it is only just past its infancy. Until the 1950s, the international perfume market was completely dominated by French fragrances. Only perfume from Paris seemed to impart the right flair, the true original elegance and exclusiveness that promised *haute couture* in a bottle.

In the end, it was not an American fashion designer who broke the French supremacy, but a woman from the cosmetics industry: Estée Lauder.

MARKETING GENIUS

Lauder's career fits the American Dream. Esther Mentzer, a young girl of Hungarian descent, from the New York area of Queens, worked as a beautician in a beauty parlour. Her uncle, a 'skin doctor', taught her how to make skin creams. With his help, she

Above: In creating her fragrances, Estée Lauder uses ingredients from around the world. 'A perfume is like a dress. It makes you feel simply marvellous.'

Right: Youth Dew, launched in 1953, was the foundation of Estée Lauder's world-wide business.

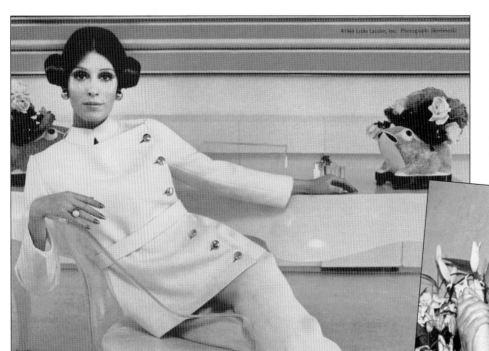

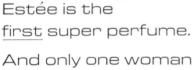

Estée is the
first super perfume.
And only one woman
could have created it.

Estée Lauder

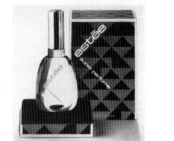

Left: Estée was launched in 1968. Its advertising reflected the philosophy of women's self-confidence, luxury and erotic elegance that is true of Estée Lauder products today.

Below: Estée Lauder's son, Leonhard, celebrates with Elizabeth Hurley – the new face of the Estée Lauder Company.

developed four different skin-care products, which she successfully tried out on her customers. As a result, she made the decision to launch her own cosmetics company with her husband, Joseph Lauder, in 1946. The company was named Estée Lauder.

Two years later, Lauder began supplying cosmetics to the exclusive New York department store *Saks*. It was here that she put into effect her first innovative marketing idea: with every cream sold, she gave away an item of toiletry as a free gift. This was unheard of in a department store like *Saks* and Estée Lauder became famous overnight.

Her cosmetics company, however, could still not compete with the leading American companies – Revlon, Helena Rubinstein and Elizabeth Arden – who had already introduced perfumes to the market. Estée Lauder decided to follow suit and create a fragrance of her own.

Perfume was still extremely expensive, a luxury article that very few women could afford. Only on special occasions would they discreetly dab perfume behind each ear, and this perfume invariably came from France.

GIFTS OF LOVE

There was another, much bigger problem. Perfume had traditionally been regarded as a romantic present from a man to a woman. In fact, women hardly dared to go out and buy perfume for themselves. 'It was considered

PROFILE

Estée Lauder

1946	The company Estée Lauder is born.
1948	First sales in the New York department store, Saks.
1960	Expansion into international markets.
1964	Start of the brand name *Aramis*. The first scent for men is launched.
1968	Start of the brand name *Clinique*.
1979	Start of the brand name *Prescriptives*.
1984	Estée Lauder wins 'Mother of the Year' award in the USA.
1990	Start of the brand name *Origins*.
1995	Actress Elizabeth Hurley becomes new top model for Estée Lauder.
1995	Estée Lauder enters the stock market.

PERFUME CHRONOLOGY

1953	*Youth Dew*	**1978**	*Cinnabar*	**1995**	*Tuscany per Donna*
1968	*Estée*	**1978**	*White Linen*		
1969	*Azurée*	**1985**	*Beautiful*	**1996**	*Pleasures*
1972	*Alliage*	**1988**	*Knowing*	**1997**	*White Linen Breeze*
1973	*Private Collection*	**1992**	*Spellbound*		

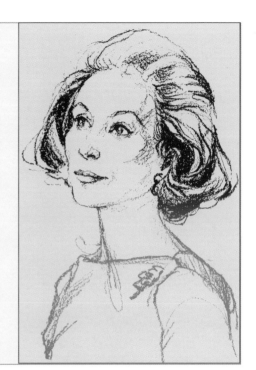

decent to wait until one was given perfume by one's fiancé – a perfume that he liked, or which he thought his lady would like,' remarked Estée Lauder.

She did her utmost to change this attitude: 'How could I get American women to buy their own perfume? I deliberately did not call it perfume, I called it *Youth Dew* – a bath oil which could also be used as perfume'. She launched *Youth Dew* in 1953, first as a bath oil and then as a perfume. Just like Guerlain's *Shalimar*, it ranks among the classic oriental fragrancies.

Youth Dew took America by storm. Within a year of its launch it secured a turnover of $50,000. Instead of dabbing drops of French perfume behind their ears, women poured bottles of *Youth Dew* into their bath water.

Another reason for the product's success may have been that, unlike the Parisian perfume makers, Estée Lauder did not seal her bottles. Customers could test the fragrance and then decide whether or not they liked it.

A PERFUME REVOLUTION

Estée Lauder's marketing practice was not only a clever way of selling her fragrance, she also believed that it helped women to gain more independence and self-confidence.

Up until then, women generally lived with one man, or husband, all their lives – and wore one scent. That had now changed. 'You wouldn't wear the same dress on the tennis court and at a party – so why wear the same perfume?' asked Estée Lauder, provocatively.

With her products, Estée Lauder triggered a small revolution that questioned the narrow morals of American society. Now Estée could allow herself to say: 'Perfume is just like love – you can never have enough of it.'

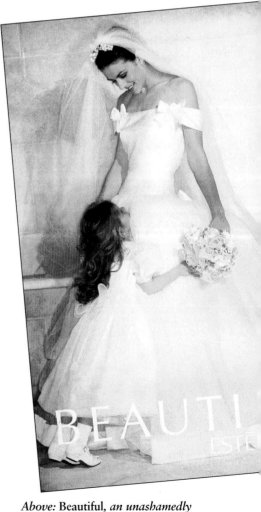

Above: Beautiful, *an unashamedly romantic fragrance, celebrated love, marriage and family.*
Right: Pleasures *has strong floral notes, giving the fragrance the scent of flowers after rain has fallen.*

Estée Lauder
COLLECTION

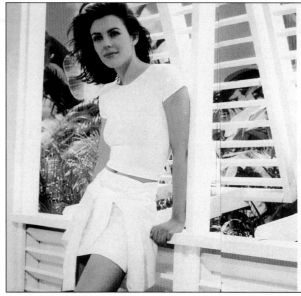

Right: Clean and crisp, with a splash of sea, sun-washed flowers and clear blue sky, White Linen Breeze *is:* 'like how a summer breeze caresses your skin on a warm summer's day.'

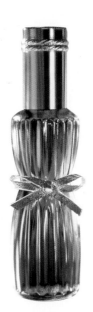

YOUTH DEW

Launch: 1953

▲ Top notes: Orange, Spices

▲ Middle notes: Clove

▲ Base note: Ambergris, Tolu

Style: A heavy, erotic, spicy oriental scent and one of the few perfumes available that is diluted in oil rather than alcohol

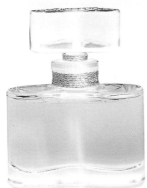

WHITE LINEN

Launch: 1978

▲ Top notes: Aldehydes

▲ Middle notes: Rose, Jasmin, Lily-of-the-valley

▲ Base notes: Cedarwood, Ambergris

Style: The classic rose-jasmin heart of this perfume exudes a warmth and sensuality that is distinctively feminine

BEAUTIFUL

Launch: 1985

▲ Top notes: Rose, Lily, Tuberose, Marigold, Cassis, Mandarin

▲ Middle notes: Jasmin, Ylang-Ylang, Orange blossom, Carnation, Thyme, Sage

▲ Base notes: Orris, Vetiver, Sandalwood, Oakmoss, Amber, Tonka, Vanilla

Style: Jasmin dominates this romantic floral fragrance and in the words of Est e Lauder is for the most beautiful moments in life.

PLEASURES

Launch: 1996

▲ Top notes: Lily, Violet leaves, Green notes

▲ Middle notes: Lilac, Peony, Rose, Baie Rose, Jasmin, Karo karounde blossom

▲ Base notes: Sandalwood, Patchouli

Style: Containing the first new natural ingredient in perfumery in 25 years — Baie Rose — *Pleasures* unfolds its scent slowly

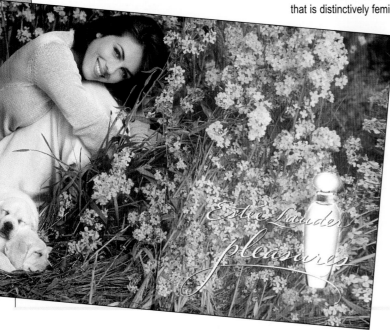
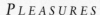
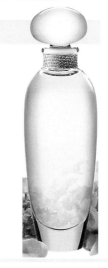
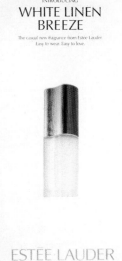

CHRISTIAN DIOR

In 1947, Christian Dior introduced the 'New Look', his first fashion collection, and became famous overnight. Today, women may no longer wear his fairytale dresses, but Dior perfumes are in more demand than ever.

Christian Dior was born in Granville, Normandy, in 1905. The son of a wealthy businessman, Dior had a carefree and happy childhood. In 1919, the family moved to Paris. Here, fascinated by theatre and modern art, Dior eagerly immersed himself in the cultural life of the city.

TROUBLED TIMES

Dior opened a gallery in Paris in 1927, together with his friend Jacques Bonhan. He exhibited works by artists such as Picasso, Léger and Chirico, who were also his good friends.

Initially, business was good, but then the world economic crisis forced the gallery to close. The crisis hit Dior's father, too, and he was forced to sell his business. To make matters worse, Christian's mother died. He fell ill and was sent to the country to recuperate.

When Dior returned to Paris, he began to design fashion, at his

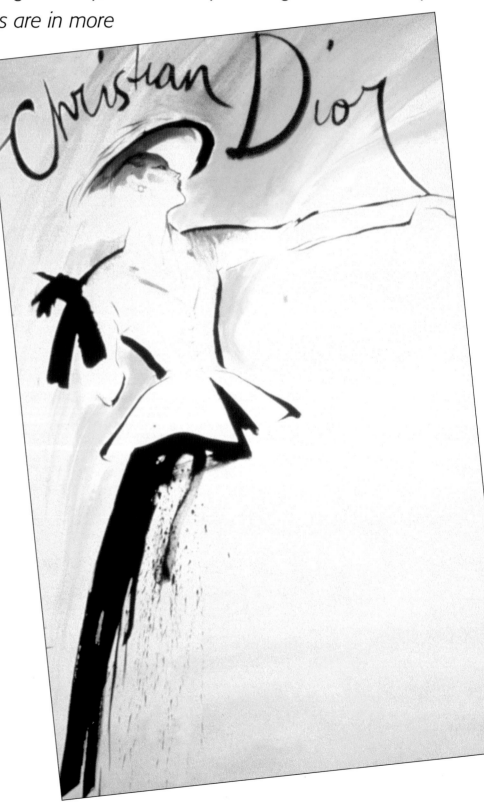

Right: Christian Dior revolutionized the fashion of the post-war years with his 'New Look'. His wasp-waist designs and whirling skirts proclaimed a femininity unseen for decades.

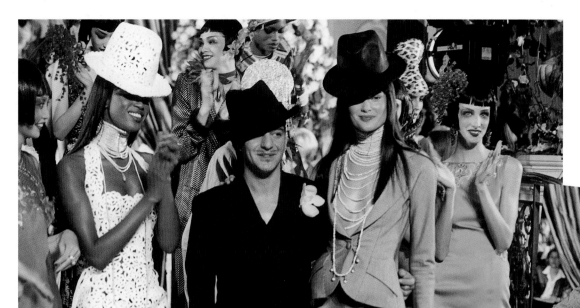

friend Jean Ozenne's insistence. To begin with, he restricted his designs to hats – just like Coco Chanel. Then, Dior's talent was discovered by the designer Robert Piguet, who employed him in 1938. World War II soon interrupted Dior's fledgling career and he spent most of the war years at the family home in the South of France.

FIRST STEPS

When Dior was able to return to Paris, a friend introduced him to the textiles magnate Marcel Boussac, who offered Dior the opportunity to open his own fashion house.

He rented a small mansion on Avenue Montaigne and had the exterior of the building painted grey and white – the colour combination which was

Right: The shape of the original Miss Dior *bottle mirrored the design of the 'New Look' fashion.*

to become his trademark in later years. The interior decoration was extremely elegant. Dior's fashion house opened on 16 December, 1946, and on 12 February, 1947, he presented his first collection, featuring the 'New Look'.

THE 'NEW LOOK'

Dior became famous overnight. After the austerity of the war years, his wasp-waisted garments, with their flowing skirts – using up to 20 metres of expensive fabric – were a revelation. They literally caused riots in the streets of Paris between those women who were for or against this seemingly wanton extravagance. The success of the 'New Look' started a 'Diormania', which Dior instantly turned into profitable business. He licensed the name *Dior*

to be used for other products, such as perfume and accessories – which resulted in the company *Parfums Christian Dior* being founded the same year.

FIRST FRAGRANCE

Dior's first fragrance was *Miss Dior,* which was sprayed in all the rooms of his fashion house, bewitching his female customers.

Christian Dior believed that fashion had to change all the time,

21

Christian Dior
COLLECTION

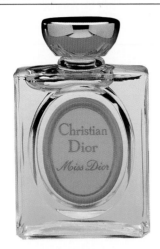

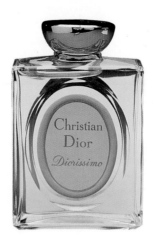

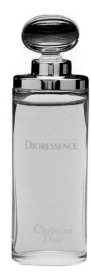

MISS DIOR

Launch: 1947
▲ Top notes: Aldehyde, Gardenia, Galbanum, Bergamot
▲ Middle notes: Jasmin, Narcissus, Rose, Orris root
▲ Base note: Patchouli, Ambergris, Vetiver, Sandalwood
Style: This flowery, animal chypre fragrance exudes a hypnotic warmth.

DIORISSIMO

Launch: 1956
▲ Top notes: Green foliage, Bergamot
▲ Middle notes: Lily-of-the-valley, Lily, Jasmin, Rose
▲ Base notes: Sandalwood, Civet
Style: *Diorissimo* has delicate fresh green top notes and the pure, direct and bewitching scent of lily-of-the-valley — Christian Dior s favourite flower.

DIORESSENCE

Launch: 1970
▲ Top notes: Aldehyde, Green notes, Orange
▲ Middle notes: Carnation, Rose, Jasmin, Cinnamon, Ylang Ylang, Orris root, Tuberose
▲ Base notes: Benzoin, Patchouli, Styrax, Vanilla, Ambergris, Musk
Style: A piquant oriental fragrance in which the aldehyd chord dominates the head notes and intensifies the oth ingredients. This perfume exudes a warmth and sensuality that is distinctively feminine.

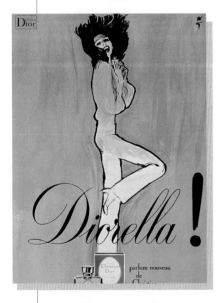

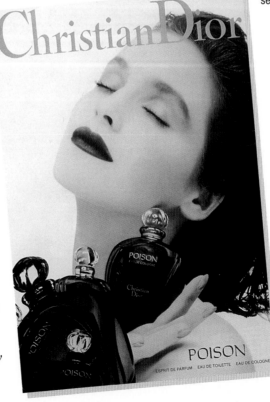

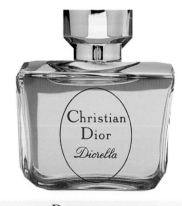

DIORELLA

Launch: 1972
▲ Top notes: Lemon, Bergamot, Melon, Basil
▲ Middle notes: Jasmin, Rose, Carnation
▲ Base notes: Oak moss, Patchouli, Vetiver, Musk
Style: The perfect match of citrus scents and green flowery notes create a light fragrance for elegant days and nights.

Above: This Diorella poster from 1972 captures the feeling and the fashion style of the disco generation.
Right: The bottle of Poison deliberately looks like some magical fruit filled with belladonna.

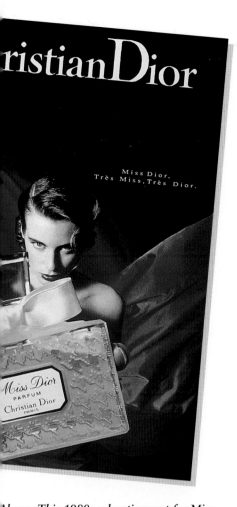

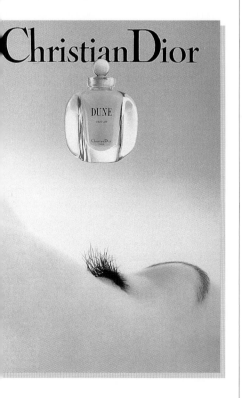

Above: This 1980s advertisement for Miss Dior *exudes a classic sophistication, as befits this feminine, very Parisian scent. Below: The marine fragrance* Dune *was launched in 1992.*

Christian Dior

1905	Christian Dior born in Granville, Normandy, France.
1938	First job as a fashion designer.
1946	Dior takes over a Paris fashion house in Avenue Montaigne.
1947	Presentation of his first collection, featuring the 'New Look'.
1957	Dior dies at the age of 52.

PERFUME CHRONOLOGY

1947	*Miss Dior*
1949	*Diorama*
1953	*Eau fraiche*
1956	*Diorissimo*
1963	*Diorling*
1966	*Eau Sauvage*
1970	*Dioressence*
1972	*Diorella*
1976	*Dior Dior*
1980	*Jules*
1984	*Eau Sauvage Extreme*
1985	*Poison*
1988	*Fahrenheit*
1991	*Dune*
1994	*Tendre Poison*
1995	*Dolce Vita*
1994	*Dune pour homme*

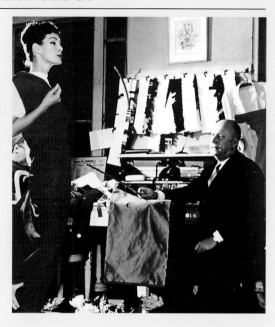

therefore he presented new creations twice a year.

Just as an artist chooses a theme for an exhibition, each one of Dior's collections had a motto. After the launch of *Miss Dior,* he began to name one of the new designs in each collection after a Dior perfume.

Few women could afford to buy Dior's clothes. The perfumes, however, were within the means of a much wider clientele. The bottles, too, conveyed pure Dior luxury, and taking part in the grand world of *haute couture.*

The perfumer Edmund Roudnitska created a new Dior fragrance in 1956. It was given the Italian-sounding name *Diorissimo* and was sold in a beautiful bottle

made of Baccarat crystal. It looked like a vase with golden roses and jasmin. Chrystiane Charles designed the gold-plated bronze flowers.

The combination of crystal and metal had been used before, but few could match the incredibly beautiful sculpture on the perfume's bottle top.

THE LEGACY

Christian Dior ranks among the most famous fashion designers of this century. When he died at the age of 52, in 1957, he left what can only be described as an empire. His legacy was his love of art, and for the past 40 years his unseen hand has guided the clothes and fragrancies created by his successors for the House of Dior.

KENZO

He is said to be the most western of the Japanese designers and the most Japanese of western designers, but he calls himself a 'flower man' – and his perfumes prove it.

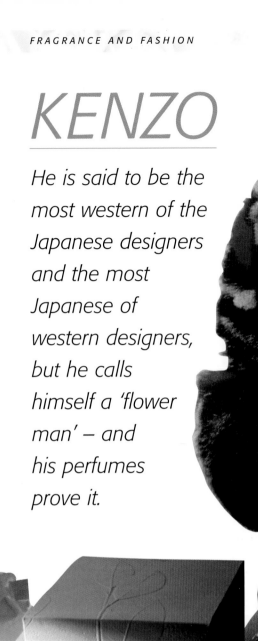

Above: Kenzo, with magnolia, gardenia and ylang-ylang, was distilled by the renowned French 'composer of scents' François Caron. The bottle was designed in the form of a pebble by the sculptor Serge Mansau.

At the beginning of 1965, a young Japanese man was strolling through the streets of Paris. He looked like one of the countless tourists, with a camera hanging around his neck, ready to snap anything that caught his eye. But he was different, not least because he had had to sell his car in Tokyo in order to get to Paris.

Above: The stylized painted faces and exuberant colours in Kenzo's 1998 collection show his continued indebtedness to traditional Japanese theatre.

The young man's name was Kenzo Takada and he was born in Himeji in 1939. Kenzo had been a prize-winning art student in Tokyo and had left, amid protests from his family and art teachers, to

Right: Kenzo, unlike most designers, supervises the making of his fragrancies.

become a fashion designer. He knew no French and had only a few francs in his pocket. But he had some of his fashion sketches with him and his first break came when the designer Louis Féraud agreed to buy five of them.

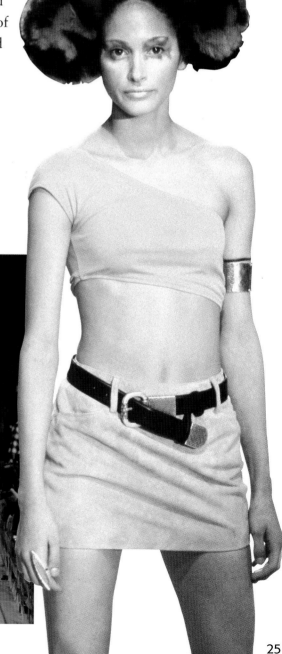

Above: Kenzo loves flowers and, as a young man, often painted them.

Below: Kenzo's recent designs have been more austere and minimalist.

WORK IN PARIS

Kenzo soon found work, first with a designer, then a textile company, and throughout the rest of the 1960s he created freelance collections. His designs were so well-received that he was able to open his own fashion boutique in 1970.

It was an immediate success, particularly after *Elle* magazine used one of his designs on its cover, reporting that Kenzo was

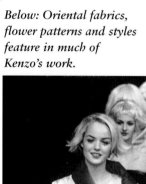

Below: Oriental fabrics, flower patterns and styles feature in much of Kenzo's work.

the most revolutionary fashion designer of the day.

COLOURFUL COTTONS

Kenzo's early cotton clothes were immensely popular, with their bright, semi-abstract floral patterns and startling colours. He was a genius at mixing prints and he used fabrics in layers, imitating oriental styles. Loose-fitting tunics, trousers and smocks were among his early trademarks.

Young people loved his fresh approach to design, which was far removed from *haute couture* and seemed to break all boundaries of class and nationality.

WORLDWIDE EMPIRE

By the mid-1970s, Kenzo had opened boutiques throughout the world and presented a collection of children's wear. In 1988, he launched his first perfume, simply called *Kenzo*, a blend of delicate oriental flowers.

More fragrances were to follow and the most recent *Jungle* collection maintains Kenzo's theme of the natural world. The flower man has, indeed, blossomed.

Right: Kenzo, launched in 1988, was a floral fragrance enriched by fruits and spices. Parfum d'été (far right) is 'the voluptuousness of flowers gorged with sun and light'.

Kenzo
C O L L E C T I O N

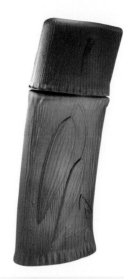

KENZO POUR HOMME

Launch: 1991
▲ Top notes: Ozone, Green foliage, Bergamot, Fennel
▲ Middle notes: Nutmeg, Clove, Sage, Geranium
▲ Base notes: Oak moss, Vetiver, Patchouli, Sandalwood, Rosewood, Musk, Iris, Cedar
Style: Kenzo s design for the bottle is based on the bamboo, a symbol of strength in his native Japan. In keeping with its aquatic feel, the fragrance is cased in blue glass with raised ribs of reed-like plants.

PARFUM D'ÉTÉ

Launch: 1992
▲ Top notes: Green notes
▲ Middle notes: Rose, Jasmin, Peony, Narcissus, Freesia, Hyacinth
▲ Base notes: Musk, Amber, Iris, Sandalwood, Oakmoss
Style: This fragrance has a harmonious, balanced bouquet, whose scent slips out lightly, like the perfume that wafts from the flowers in a garden. The summer mood it evokes lasts all year round.

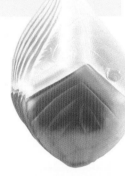

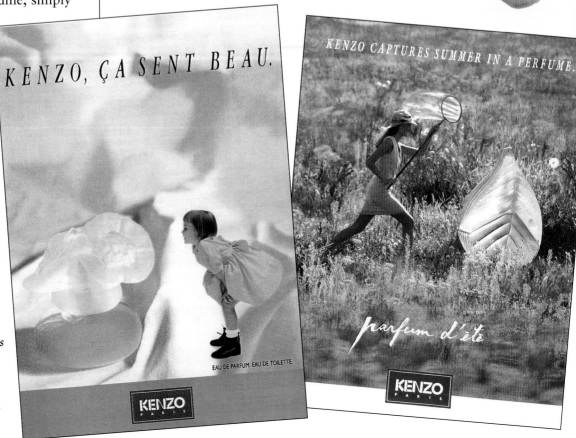

KENZO, ÇA SENT BEAU.

EAU DE PARFUM. EAU DE TOILETTE.

KENZO CAPTURES SUMMER IN A PERFUME.

parfum d'été

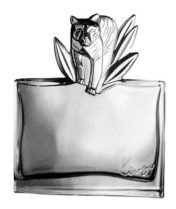

JUNGLE TIGER

Launch: 1998

▲ Top notes: Kumquat, Davana

▲ Middle notes: Chinese osmanthus, Ylang-ylang

▲ Base note: Amber, Massoia wood, Cinnamon

Style: Made from a composition of Asian spices, fruits, flowers and woods, *Jungle Tiger* provides a wild, yet mild and warm, sensuality.

L'EAU PAR KENZO

Launch: 1996

▲ Top notes: Reed stems, Mint

▲ Middle notes: Jasmin water, Paradise seed

▲ Base notes: Blue cedar, Vanilla pods

Style: The magic formula of frosted mint, jasmin water and vanilla makes a free-spirited fragrance for any time or place.

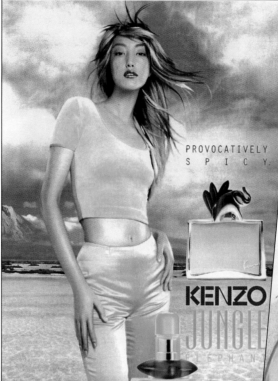

PROVOCATIVELY SPICY.

KENZO JUNGLE ELEPHANT

l'eau par Kenzo

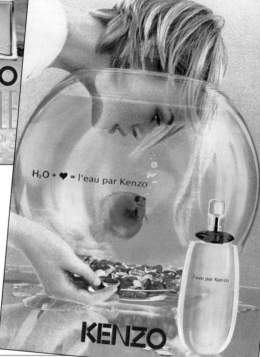

Left: Jungle Eléphant *was inspired by Kenzo's love of elephants. He has a cherished good-luck charm, in the shape of a miniature elephant, that never leaves his side.*

Below: L'eau par Kenzo *captures the freshness of water and natural scents.*

H_2O + ♥ = l'eau par Kenzo

l'eau par Kenzo

KENZO

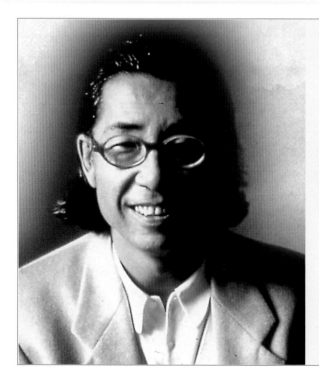

PROFILE

Kenzo

1940	Born Kenzo Takada in Himeji, Japan.
1965	Kenzo moves to Paris. Sells first designs to Louis Féraud.
1970	Opens his own shop, Jungle Jap.
1970	First collection presented in Paris.
1988	Launches first perfume, *Kenzo*.
1990	Institutes 'chair' for financing young foreign artists.
1993	Designs costumes for the opera.

PERFUME CHRONOLOGY

1988	*Kenzo*	**1996**	*Jungle Eléphant*
1991	*Kenzo pour homme*	**1997**	*Jungle Tiger*
1992	*Parfum d'été*	**1997**	*Le monde est beau*
1994	*Kashaya*	**1998**	*Jungle pour hommes*
1996	*L'eau par Kenzo*	**1998**	*Jungle Zebra*

YVES SAINT-LAURENT

With his ability to embody classicism, elegance and comfort, Yves Saint-Laurent has been the world's leading designer for 40 years.

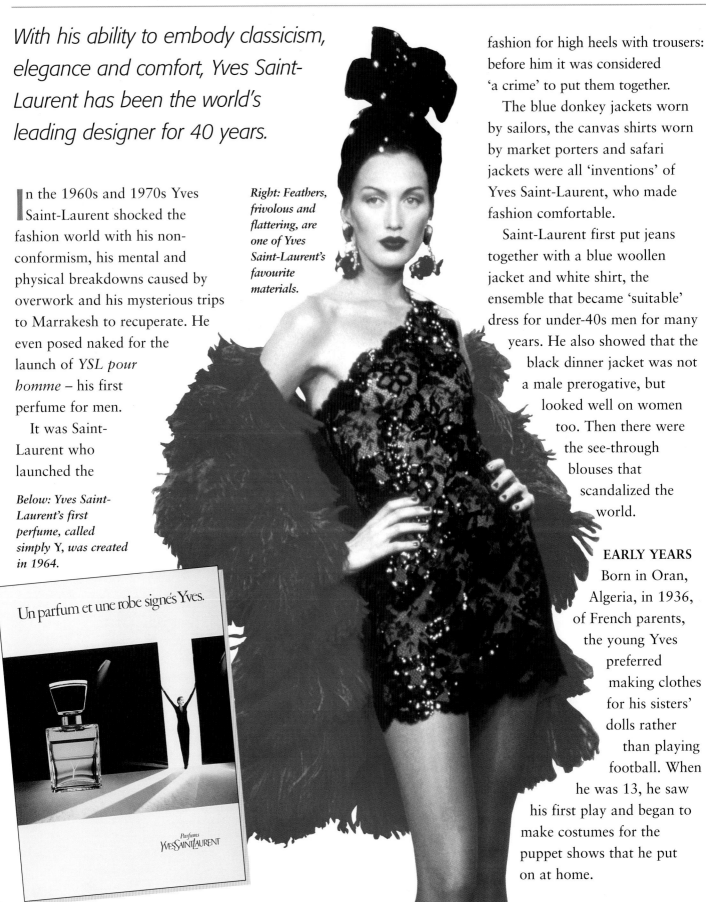

In the 1960s and 1970s Yves Saint-Laurent shocked the fashion world with his non-conformism, his mental and physical breakdowns caused by overwork and his mysterious trips to Marrakesh to recuperate. He even posed naked for the launch of *YSL pour homme* – his first perfume for men.

It was Saint-Laurent who launched the

Below: Yves Saint-Laurent's first perfume, called simply Y, was created in 1964.

Right: Feathers, frivolous and flattering, are one of Yves Saint-Laurent's favourite materials.

Un parfum et une robe signés Yves.

Parfums
YVES SAINT LAURENT

fashion for high heels with trousers: before him it was considered 'a crime' to put them together.

The blue donkey jackets worn by sailors, the canvas shirts worn by market porters and safari jackets were all 'inventions' of Yves Saint-Laurent, who made fashion comfortable.

Saint-Laurent first put jeans together with a blue woollen jacket and white shirt, the ensemble that became 'suitable' dress for under-40s men for many years. He also showed that the black dinner jacket was not a male prerogative, but looked well on women too. Then there were the see-through blouses that scandalized the world.

EARLY YEARS
Born in Oran, Algeria, in 1936, of French parents, the young Yves preferred making clothes for his sisters' dolls rather than playing football. When he was 13, he saw his first play and began to make costumes for the puppet shows that he put on at home.

Later, he studied at the local Art Academy but always hoped to go to France. When he found a newspaper announcement from the Secretariat for Wool saying that they were looking for new talent for the fashion world, Yves sent a design for a black cocktail dress and won first prize.

ASSISTANT TO DIOR

As soon as the 19-year-old Yves arrived in Paris, he enrolled in a cutting and sewing course. In the meantime, the editor of *Vogue*, Michel de Brunhoff, saw some of his sketches and realized they bore an astonishing resemblance to those of the A-line that Christian Dior was working on in secret. He spoke to Dior and arranged a meeting. A few days later, Yves Saint-Laurent joined Dior as his first assistant.

Christian Dior died suddenly two years later, but Saint-Laurent had already learned a great deal

Right: Wedding gowns are always the last display of an Yves Saint-Laurent fashion show. Here Claudia Schiffer plays the bride in the Paris show of spring 1997.

Below: Yves Saint-Laurent is photographed with his models at the autumn-winter ready-to-wear show of 1994. From left to right they are: Linda Evangelista, Maayou Keret and Karen Mulder.

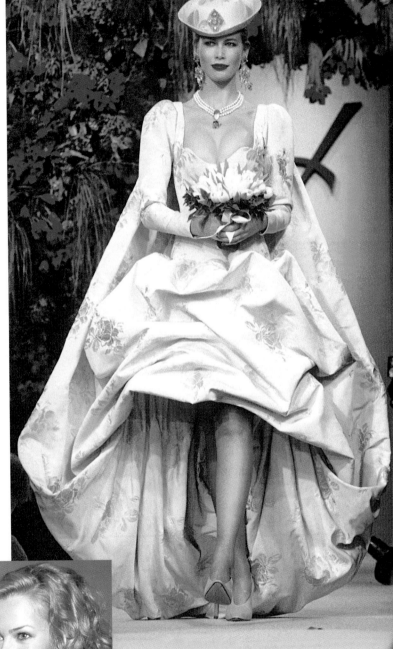

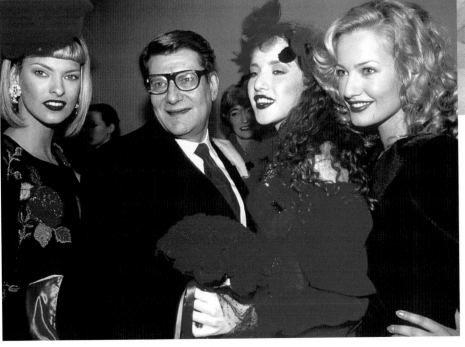

and at 21 was appointed chief designer at Dior. He was a tremendous success. As a result of his first collections, Dior found itself exporting almost 50 per cent of French designer clothing. But in 1960 Yves had to do military service. Afterwards he found himself at a crossroads: should he go back to working for Dior or open his own fashion business? He chose to set up his own company with his friend Pierre Bergé, with the American cosmetics company Charles of the Ritz providing the capital. His first highly successful fashion show was in 1962 and *Y*, his first perfume, was launched two years later.

THE SMELL OF SUCCESS
In 1966 Saint-Laurent opened his ready-to-wear boutique Rive Gauche, which gave its name to his second perfume. Launched in 1971, *Rive Gauche* was a toilet

water aimed at younger women. Instead of the classic bottle for the bathroom shelf, it was a simple spray in a blue-black canister which could be taken anywhere.

The scandalous *Opium* followed in 1977; *Paris*, his tribute to his adopted home and the rose, in 1983; and a further creation, *Yvresse légère*, in 1997. Yet although his clothes blend elegance and comfort, and his fragrances whisper romantic freedom, Yves Saint-Laurent still claims that: 'A man or a woman's most beautiful adornment is love.'

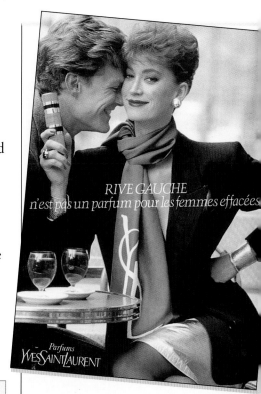

Above: Rive Gauche, *launched in 1971, was designed for the modern woman.*
Below: Opium, *with its provocative name and classic oriental bottle, shocked the world when it was launched in 1977.*

PROFILE

Yves Saint-Laurent

1936	Yves Saint-Laurent born in Oran, Algeria.
1954	Moves to Paris to attend design school run by the Chambre Syndicale de la Haute Couture. Joins Christian Dior as his first assistant.
1957	After Dior's death, Saint-Laurent is chosen as his successor.
1961	Founds his own fashion house.
1962	Presents his first collection under his own name.
1966	Opens his first ready-to-wear boutique, Rive Gauche.
1968	Yves Saint-Laurent creates the 'Safari' look.
1971	Launch of his fragrance *Rive Gauche*.
1982	Receives the International Award of the Council of Fashion Designers of America.
1983	Metropolitan Museum of Art in New York holds exhibition – the first for a living designer.
1986	Appointed as a senior adviser to the People's Republic of China.
1992	Thirtieth anniversary of Yves Saint-Laurent fashion house.

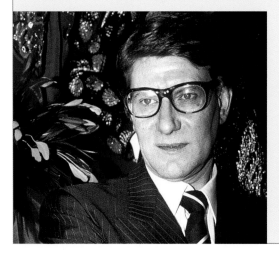

PERFUME CHRONOLOGY

1964	*Y*
1971	*Rive Gauche*
1971	*YSL pour homme*
1975	*Eau libre*
1977	*Opium*
1981	*Kouros pour homme*
1983	*Paris*
1993	*Champagne*
1995	*Opium pour homme*
1997	*Yvresse*
1997	*Yvresse légère*

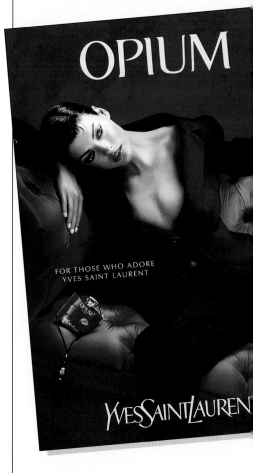

OPIUM

FOR THOSE WHO ADORE
YVES SAINT LAURENT

Yves Saint-Laurent
C O L L E C T I O N

RIVE GAUCHE

Launch: 1971

▲ Top notes: Ylang-ylang, Jasmin, Rose, Gardenia, Aldehyde

▲ Middle notes: Sandalwood

▲ Base notes: Lemon

Style: A 1970s classic that was designed for women more interested in style than fashion, this fragrance is for outdoor living and travel, echoed by its metallic go-anywhere canister.

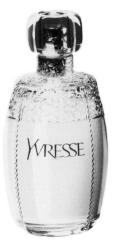

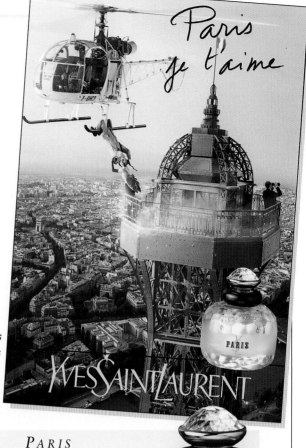

Right: Paris *was Saint-Laurent's tribute to the rose.*

OPIUM

Launch: 1977

▲ Top notes: Tangerine

▲ Middle notes: Myrrh, Jasmin

▲ Base notes: Vanilla

Style: Oriental, spicy, fruity and floral, *Opium* evokes the softness of sunkissed fruits and spices.

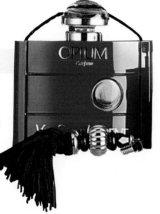

PARIS

Launch: 1983

▲ Top notes: Damask rose, Grasse rose, Hawthorn, Bergamot, Juniper berry

▲ Middle notes: Violet, Carnation, Mimosa, Honey

▲ Base notes: Vetiver, Amber, Musk

Style: This unashamedly floral fragrance, with its heady mixture of all kinds of rose petals and spring blooms, is the most beautiful fragrance in the world.

YVRESSE LÉGÈRE

Launch: 1997

▲ Top notes: Nectarine flower, Mint, Blackcurrant leaves

▲ Middle notes: Blue rose, Mimosa, White lilac

▲ Base notes: Vetiver, Oakmoss, Patchouli

Style: A fresh, lively fragrance in a bold modern style.

Right: Yvresse *is a play on words. In French* ivresse *means a state of intoxication.*

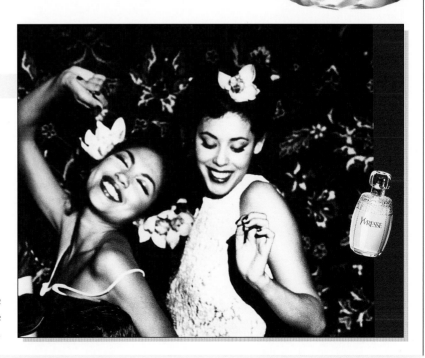

CALVIN KLEIN

The clothes and fragrances produced by Calvin Klein over the last 30 years reflect his own extraordinary odyssey through the American Dream.

One spring day in 1969, the vice-president of the New York department store Bonwit Teller pressed the wrong button in the lift of the York Hotel and found himself in the workroom of a struggling freelance coat designer. Impressed by the samples he saw, he invited the young man to show them to his store buyer. The following day, Calvin Klein

Right: Stella Tennant models a schoolgirl tunic dress from Klein's autumn 1997 collection.

Below: Calvin Klein has produced male versions of many of his fragrances.

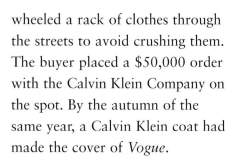

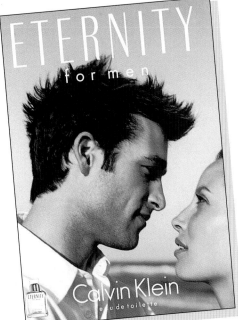

wheeled a rack of clothes through the streets to avoid crushing them. The buyer placed a $50,000 order with the Calvin Klein Company on the spot. By the autumn of the same year, a Calvin Klein coat had made the cover of *Vogue*.

RAGS TO RICHES

Klein's is an archetypal American rags-to-riches story. The son of a Bronx grocer, he worked his way through art school, then set up his own company with $10,000 lent by a childhood friend, Bernie Schwarz – still his business partner. He now heads a huge international corporation that designs, makes, sells, distributes or licenses everything from *haute couture* to jeans, fragrances to underwear, and spectacles to swimwear. The perfume business alone generates sales of over $500 million a year.

Like all fairytales, Klein's has its darker moments. His first marriage collapsed, and in 1978 he had to pay kidnappers a ransom for his young daughter, Marci. He was part of the Manhattan jetset that partied the nights away at clubs, such as Studio 54, and succumbed temporarily to the twin lures of cocaine and alcohol before sobering up.

A TALENT FOR RENEWAL

Klein has a talent – bordering on genius – for turning setbacks to his advantage, and for reinventing

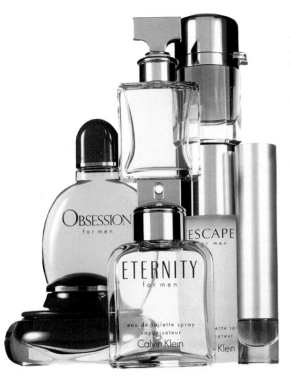

Left: Since the launch of Obsession *in 1985, Calvin Klein has built up an impressive range of fragrances.*

Right: Kate Moss, one of Klein's favourite models, wears a simply-cut, unadorned satin gown in his 1998 collection.

Below: Klein is seen here with some of his models on a promotional visit to London.

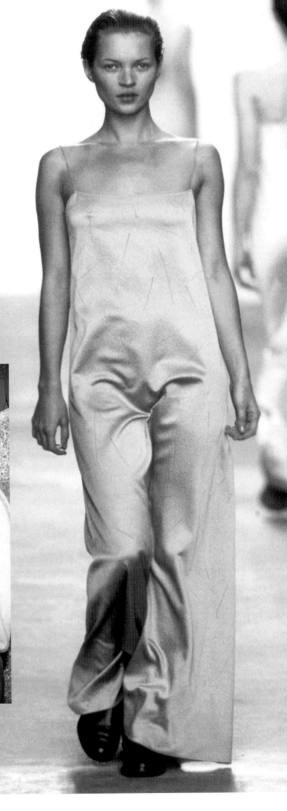

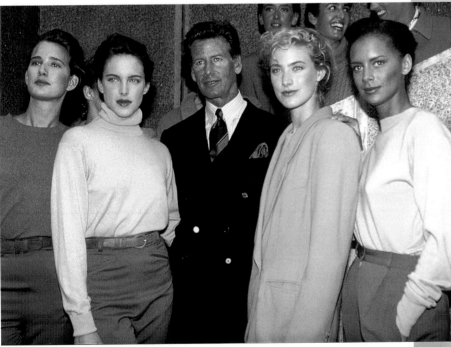

himself and his products in the spirit of the times. In the 1970s his clothes were described as 'disco chic'; in the 1980s the clothes – and the advertisements – encapsulated the go-getting, materialistic outlook of the yuppies; and in the 1990s they expressed a softer, more homespun mood, with family, country pursuits and the healthy outdoor life being featured.

DESIGN PHILOSOPHY

His design philosophy is simple: 'Everything begins with the cut.' Throughout his career he has used high-quality, wonderfully tactile fabrics – silk, pure wool, camel, cashmere, linen and cotton – to make clothes that are both classy and understated. They are casual, sporty and easy to wear, but with a feeling of luxury. Except for a brief flirtation with grunge in the early 1990s, his designs have always been classic rather than gimmicky, but they are also young, dynamic and distinctively American.

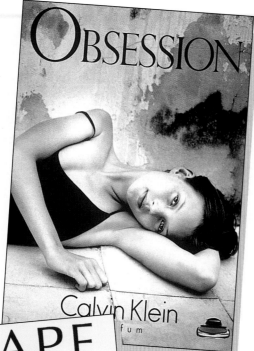

Calvin Klein
C O L L E C T I O N

OBSESSION (FOR WOMEN)

Launch date: 1985

▲ Top notes: Mandarin, Bergamot, Vanilla, Green notes
▲ Middle notes: Jasmin, Orange blossom, Sandalwood, Vetiver, Coriander, Tagette, Basil
▲ Base notes: Amber, Oakmoss, Incense, Musk
Style: This intoxicating oriental blend of florals and spices with an earthy warm base is intensely feminine and lingering. The bottle, with its mock tortoiseshell cap, was designed by Pierre Dinand, and inspired by the Kleins collection of Indian prayer stones.

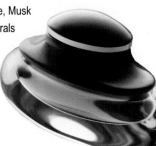

ETERNITY (FOR WOMEN)

Launch: 1988

▲ Top notes: Freesia, Mandarin, Sage
▲ Middle notes: Lily-of-the-valley, White lily, Marigold, Narcissus
▲ Base notes: Patchouli, Sandalwood, Amber
Style: Inspired by Calvin Klein s marriage to Kelly Rector (from whom he separated in 1998), and by the diamond eternity ring, once owned by the Duchess of Windsor, that he gave her, this is a romantic blend of delicate flower scents with a warm exotic edge of spices and sandalwood.

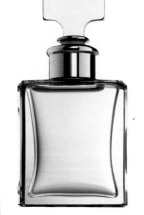

In the 1970s he launched his 'designer jeans' – the ultimate in casual chic. He and photographer Richard Avedon conceived a sensational campaign featuring the young Brooke Shields declaring that 'Nothing comes between me and my Calvin's', introducing overt sexuality into fashion promotion.

COURTING CONTROVERSY
The company's marketing of both perfume and fashion have set out to court controversy. Giant billboards of men in Calvin Klein underwear stopped traffic in New York's streets, and in 1985 the *New York Times* refused to run risqué ads for *Obsession*, which launched Klein's new fragrance company. When the waif-like Kate Moss posed nude for a perfume ad, Klein was accused of promoting anorexia and paedophilia, but the louder the protests the more sales soared.

Like his clothes, the fragrances have mirrored developments in Klein's life. *Obsession* symbolized the feverish intensity of living for the moment, and *Eternity* expressed his commitment to his new wife Kelly Rector. *Escape* reflected a new yearning for the simple life, away from the glamour of the city.

Klein's clothes often have an androgynous quality; in the ads, male and female bodies may be indistinguishable. The unisex *CK one* expresses his fascination with the blurring of genders. *CK be* and *Contradiction*, his latest fragrances, are two further intriguing stages in the evolution of this extraordinary chameleon.

CK ONE

Launch: 1994

▲ Top notes: Bergamot, Cardamom, Pineapple, Papaya
▲ Middle notes: Hedione High Cis (a special formula derived from jasmin), Violet, Rose, Nutmeg
▲ Base notes: Musk, Amber, Oakmoss

Style: The first male-female fragrance to be released in some time, this is a chypre-style perfume — light, bright, fruity and sensual, with a warm woody base. Clean and refreshing, it is meant to be splashed on liberally, both day and night. The bottle is designed by Fabien Baron, art director of *Harper s Bazaar* in New York and designer of Madonna s notorious book *Sex*.

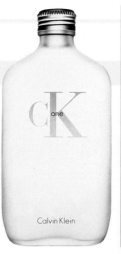

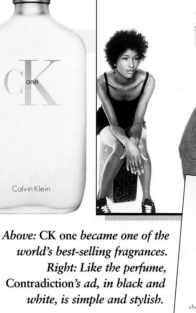

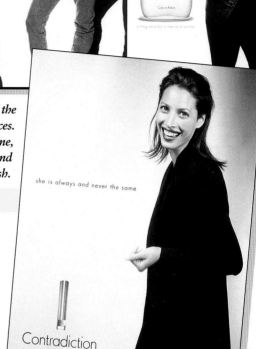

Above: CK one *became one of the world's best-selling fragrances. Right: Like the perfume,* Contradiction's *ad, in black and white, is simple and stylish.*

CONTRADICTION (FOR WOMEN)

Launch: 1998

▲ Top notes: Chinese eucalyptus, Pepper flower, White lilac, To-Yo-Ran orchid
▲ Middle notes: Lily-of-the-valley, Jasmin, Old roses, Peony
▲ Base notes: Tambouti wood, Tonka, Satinwood, Sandalwood

Style: This is a complex, provocative, oriental-style fragrance for the modern woman, who is always but never the same . Like all Klein s bottles, the silver cylinder, with just a show of amber liquid, is unusual, extremely simple and very chic.

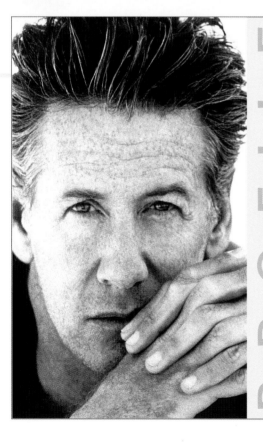

Calvin Klein

PROFILE

1942	Calvin Klein born in the Bronx, New York City, USA.
1962	Graduates from New York Fashion Insitute of Technology.
1968	Starts own company with Bernie Schwarz.
1975	Becomes first designer to win the Coty American Critics Fashion Award three years running.
1978	Launches 'designer jeans' with the Brooke Shields campaign conceived by Richard Avedon.
1985	Launch of first fragrance, *Obsession*.
1986	Marries Kelly Rector.
1991	Company reorganized into design and licensing rather than manufacture.
1993	Voted Designer of the Year for womenswear and menswear by the Council of Fashion Designers of America, the first designer to receive both awards in the same year.
1994	Launches unisex perfume *CK one*.

PERFUME CHRONOLOGY

1985	*Obsession*	1993	*Escape for men*
1986	*Obsession for men*	1994	*CK one*
1988	*Eternity*	1997	*CK be*
1989	*Eternity for men*	1998	*Contradiction for women*
1991	*Escape*	1998	*Contradiction for men*

BENETTON

Like the company's brightly coloured, cheerful clothes, Benetton fragrances are well made, light-hearted, uncomplicated and fun to wear.

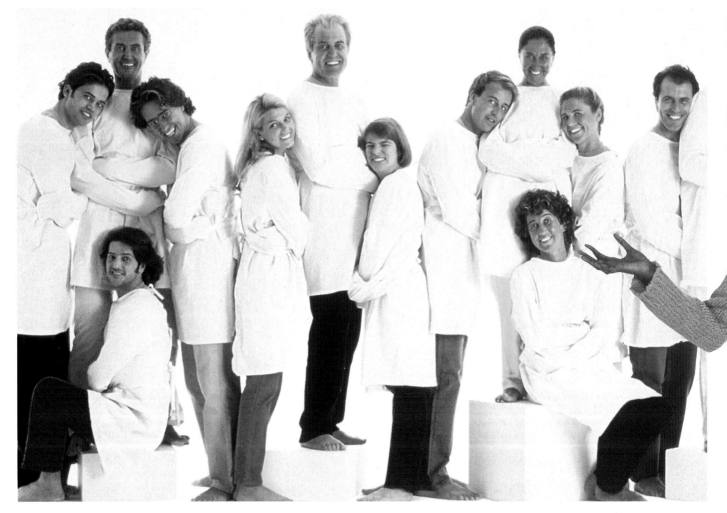

Above: Carlo, Gilberto and Giuliana Benetton (back, left to right) are pictured here with some of their staff.

It is rare that a fashion company is known as much for its sensational advertising and promotion as for its clothes. In fact, in Benetton ads, masterminded by Milanese art director and photographer Oliviero Toscani, the clothes are frequently nowhere to be seen. Instead, there are controversial, sometimes brutally realist, images of newborn babies, a dying AIDS patient, famine in Africa and a priest and nun kissing.

Their supporters say the ads break taboos and help to promote tolerance and anti-racism; others say they are hypocritical, just meant to attract attention in an image-saturated world.

HIT PROMOTIONS

Toscani invented the slogan 'United Colors of Benetton', and his first hit campaign 'All the Colors of the World' came soon after he joined the company in 1983. It featured a multiracial line-up of children dressed in the kind of brightly coloured, easy-to-wear separates that had been Benetton's stock-in-trade since its foundation.

Started in 1965 with one shop in Ponzano, near Treviso in northern Italy, by the three Benetton brothers, Carlo, Gilberto and Luciano (president) and sister

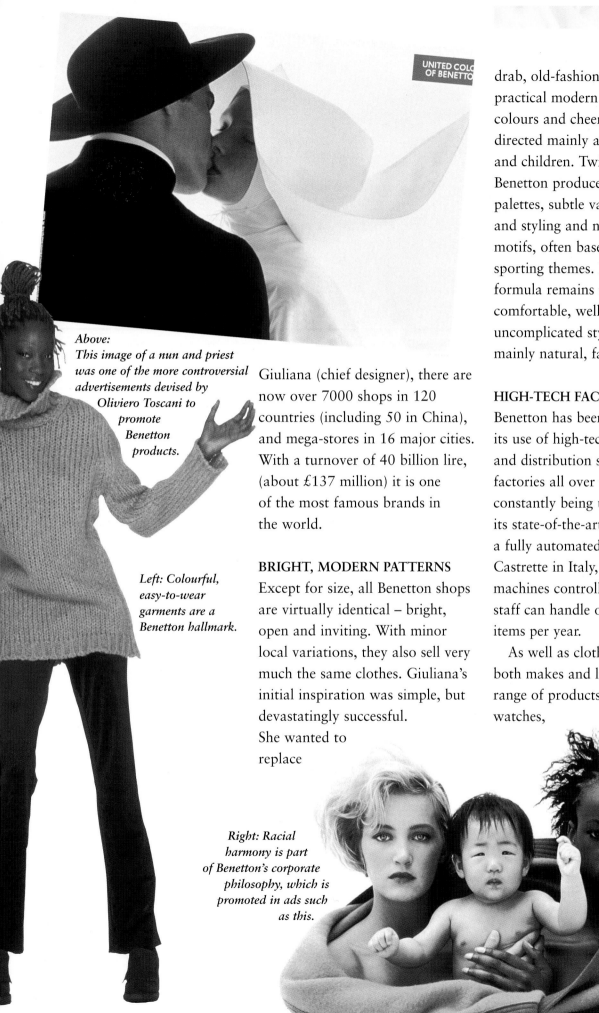

drab, old-fashioned knitwear with practical modern styles in bright colours and cheerful patterns directed mainly at young people and children. Twice a year Benetton produces new colour palettes, subtle variations on shape and styling and new pattern motifs, often based on ethnic or sporting themes. But the basic formula remains the same: comfortable, well-cut, uncomplicated styles in good, mainly natural, fabrics.

Above:
This image of a nun and priest was one of the more controversial advertisements devised by Oliviero Toscani to promote Benetton products.

Giuliana (chief designer), there are now over 7000 shops in 120 countries (including 50 in China), and mega-stores in 16 major cities. With a turnover of 40 billion lire, (about £137 million) it is one of the most famous brands in the world.

HIGH-TECH FACTORIES
Benetton has been progressive in its use of high-tech manufacturing and distribution systems. Its factories all over the world are constantly being updated, and in its state-of-the-art Robostore 2000, a fully automated warehouse at Castrette in Italy, giant robotic machines controlled by just 19 staff can handle over 100 million items per year.

Left: Colourful, easy-to-wear garments are a Benetton hallmark.

BRIGHT, MODERN PATTERNS
Except for size, all Benetton shops are virtually identical – bright, open and inviting. With minor local variations, they also sell very much the same clothes. Giuliana's initial inspiration was simple, but devastatingly successful.
She wanted to replace

As well as clothing, Benetton both makes and licenses a huge range of products: cosmetics, toys, watches,

Right: Racial harmony is part of Benetton's corporate philosophy, which is promoted in ads such as this.

Benetton

PROFILE

1965 The company is founded near Treviso, northern Italy, by the Benetton siblings – Luciano (b.1935), Giuliana (b.1938), Gilberto (b.1941) and Carlo (b.1943).

1968 First Benetton shop opens in Ponzano, Italy.

1978 Begins major European expansion campaign.

1979 First US outlet opened in New York.

1983 Becomes involved with Formula One racing.

1983 Photographer Oliviero Toscani hired to mastermind Benetton's advertising strategy.

1984 Toscani launches first hit advertising campaign: 'Benetton – All the Colors of the World'.

1985 Slogan 'United Colors of Benetton' is born.

1987 Launches first perfume *Colors*.

1994 Toscani wins Art Directors' Club Award for his work with Benetton.

PERFUME CHRONOLOGY

1987 *Colors*

1988 *Colors Uomo*

1993 *Tribù* (Luciano Benetton at its launch, right)

1994 *Hot*

1994 *Cold*

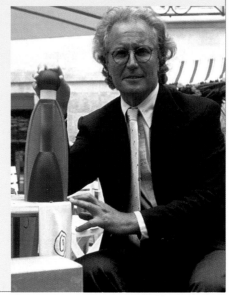

spectacles, stationery, swimwear and shoes. Benetton also invests in its local Italian sporting teams, and has a long-term involvement in Formula One racing.

In this family firm turned global empire, Benetton's perfumes play a relatively minor role. But the five fragrances in the repertoire – *Colors, Colors Uomo, Tribù* and *Hot* and *Cold* – perfectly reflect the corporate philosophy: youthful, cheerful, light-hearted and fun. They are uncomplicated, everyday fragrances, cleverly packaged and good value for money.

Left: This knitwear item appeared in Benetton's winter collection of 1997/98.

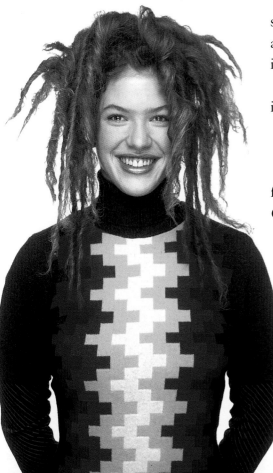

Benetton

COLLECTION

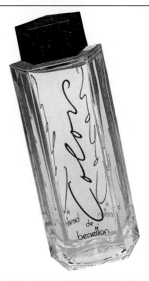

COLORS

Launch: 1987

▲ Top notes: Bergamot, Mandarin, Green notes, Violet, Melon, Marigold

▲ Middle notes: Jasmin, Tuberose, Hyacinth, Rose, Ylang-ylang, Lily-of-the-valley

▲ Base notes: Cedar, Sandalwood, Amber, Musk, Moss, Vanilla

Style: The name and multi-coloured packaging of Benetton s first fragrance reflect the corporate identity, and its identification with youth and global themes. The perfume is light, fresh and flowery, fleshed out with warm notes of spice and precious woods.

HOT

Launch: 1997

▲ Top notes: Citrus fruit

▲ Middle notes: Rosewood, Jasmin, Apricot

▲ Base notes: Sandalwood, Vanilla

Style: As relaxing as a warm bath after a hectic day, this is a lightly floral unisex perfume with the slight tang of citrus. The *Hot* and *Cold* fragrances are intended to be used as liberally as water (hence the tap-shaped screwtops in red for *Hot* and blue for *Cold*).

COLORS UOMO

Launch: 1988

▲ Top notes: Green notes, Bergamot, Lemon, Lavender, Tarragon, Coriander

▲ Middle notes: Cypress, Pine, Cyclamen, Jasmin, Carnation, Rose, Fern

▲ Base notes: Vanilla, Benzoin, Cedar, Patchouli, Sandalwood, Amber

Style: An oriental-style male fragrance, which is fresh, exhilarating and tangy but with flowery resinous undertones.

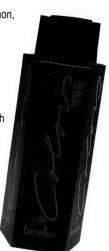

COLORS, PERFUME OF THE WORLD.

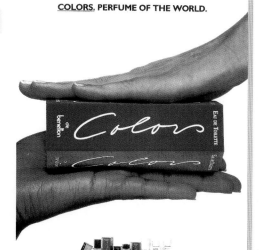

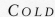

Left: This striking ad for Colors, *Benetton's first fragrance, highlights its clever packaging, as well as the range of toiletries in which it is used.*

TRIBÙ

Launch: 1993

▲ Top notes: Cassis, Marigold, Peach, Camomile, Galbanum, Violet

▲ Middle notes: Geranium, Ylang-ylang, Rose, Jasmin, Iris, Jacaranda wood

▲ Base notes: Sandalwood, Vetiver, Oakmoss, Benzoin, Tonka bean

Style: A warm, light-hearted, floral-fruity perfume with soft, dusty, woody notes, it uses no animal products or synthetics and no animal testing was involved in its manufacture.

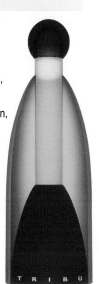

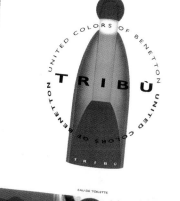

Right: Tribù *contains exotic ingredients from East and West, as its advertising suggests.*

Below: Multiracial images are a feature of many Benetton ads.

COLD

Launch: 1997

▲ Top notes: Bergamot, Mandarin, Neroli, Lavender, Verbena

▲ Middle notes: Thyme, Coriander, Geranium

▲ Base notes: Patchouli, Vetiver, White moss, Amber

Style: As invigorating as a cold shower, and a companion to *Hot*, this is a fresh, sharp chypre-style fragrance — lively and energetic, and full of youthful vitality.

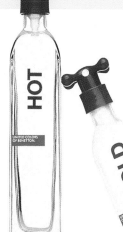

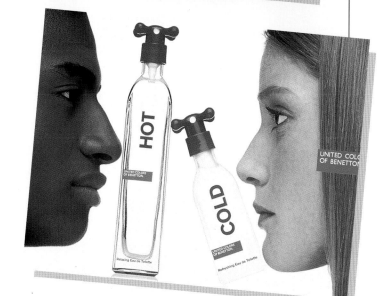

GIVENCHY

Tall, handsome and courteous, Hubert de Givenchy came to be known as 'the perfect gentleman of couture', a byword for elegance and simplicity.

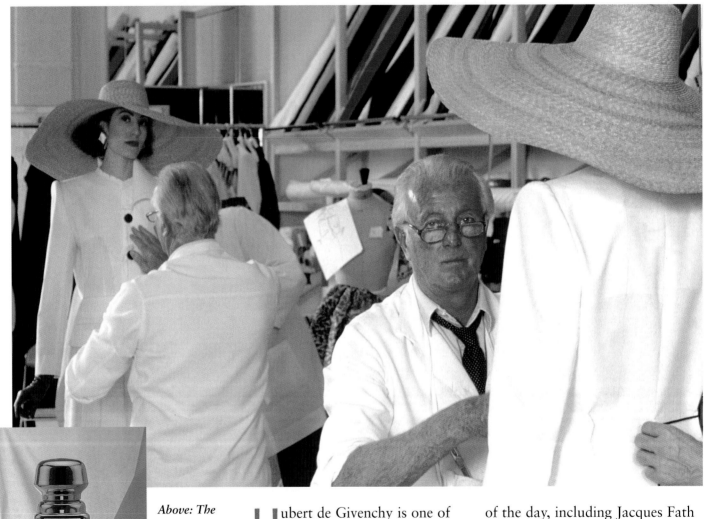

Above: The Givenchy house style is a graceful minimalism, expressed in simple lines and fine fabrics with few or no decorative flourishes.

Hubert de Givenchy is one of the great names in French fashion, the epitome of refinement and elegance. His designs have adorned the most glamorous women of the century, including Princess Grace, the Duchess of Windsor and Jacqueline Onassis.

He studied at the Ecole des Beaux Arts in Paris, and worked with some of the hottest designers

Left: The stylish image of fragrances such as Givenchy III expresses the same effortless elegance as Givenchy's couture.

of the day, including Jacques Fath and Elsa Schiaparelli, but his idol was Balenciaga, who became a life-long friend and mentor. The year they met, 1953, was a turning point for Givenchy in other ways: his first collection proved an immediate success and he met Audrey Hepburn, whom he would transform from a girlish gamine into the embodiment of womanly style and sophistication. In return, she remained his muse and ardent supporter all her life.

40

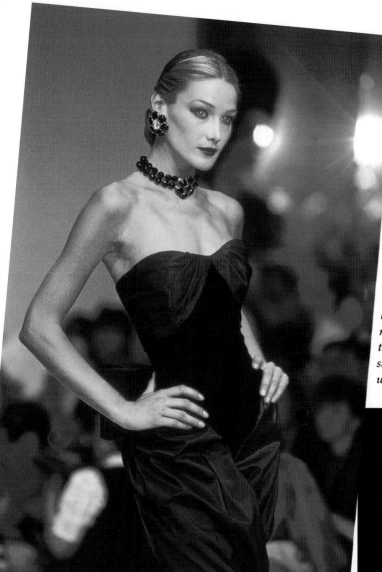

Above: Givenchy's last collection before his retirement in 1995 maintained his hallmarks of elegance and simplicity. This classic black evening gown is modelled by Carla Bruni.

Below: None of Hubert de Givenchy's glamorous clients excited his imagination in the same way as Audrey Hepburn, whom he saw as his muse. She, in turn, believed she 'was born to wear his clothes'.

such as *Sabrina*, *Funny Face* and *Breakfast at Tiffany's*.

In the 1980s, Givenchy turned to street fashion for inspiration, rekindling his early passion for extravagance and pattern. After he retired, the young British designers John Galliano and Alexander McQueen were successively appointed chief designer, adding a fresh, experimental verve to the refined traditions of Givenchy.

Givenchy Parfums was launched in 1957 with two fragrances, *Le de Givenchy* and *L'Interdit*, the latter dedicated to Audrey

Givenchy's early clothes were youthful and exuberant, focusing on luxurious separates in cheerful prints and imaginatively embroidered fabrics. His later designs, strongly influenced by Balenciaga, were simpler and more restrained. Together the two men launched the 'sack' dress – a loose chemise tapering from shoulders to hem.

ESSENTIAL GIVENCHY

By the early 1960s, the essential Givenchy house style had evolved: classically elegant clothes, formal but feminine – the kind of clothes worn by Audrey Hepburn in films

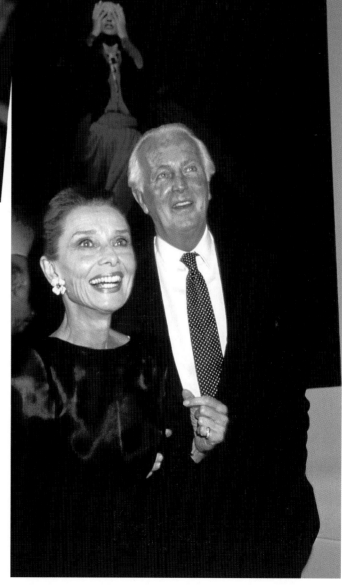

Givenchy
COLLECTION

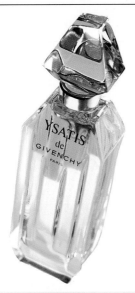

YSATIS

Launch: 1984
▲ Top notes: Mandarin, Ylang-ylang
▲ Middle notes: Jasmin, Egyptian rose, Florentine iris, Orange blossom
▲ Base notes: Vanilla, Sandalwood, Clove, Precious woods, Amber
Style: This is a classic chypre-style blend of over 100 notes, which combines the richness of oriental spices and precious woods with the heady sensuality of exotic blossom. It is still one of the world s top-selling perfumes.

AMARIGE

Launch: 1991
▲ Top notes: Tangerine, Violet, Rosewood
▲ Middle notes: Gardenia, Mimosa, Red fruits, Ylang-ylang
▲ Base notes: Ambergris, Precious woods, Musk, Vanilla
Style: The soft floral notes mix with sun-ripened fruit to make an exuberant blend of tangy freshness and gentle sweetness. Sensuous woody base notes provide its distinctive vitality.

Right: Givenchy described Amarige as 'a delightfully feminine fragrance evoking all the excitement and joie de vivre of youth'.

Below right: The advertising for Organza promoted cool elegance, while the launch campaign for Extravagance d'Amarige projected a more direct, raunchier image.

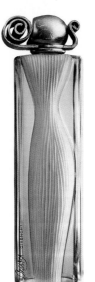

ORGANZA

Launch: 1996
▲ Top notes: Honeysuckle, Green notes
▲ Middle notes: Gardenia, Ylang-ylang, Tuberose
▲ Base notes: Vanilla, Iris, Mace, Nutmeg, Cedar, Guaiacum wood, Sandalwood, Amber
Style: The most popular of Givenchy s fragrances, *Organza* has an immediate, sappy, floral freshness and a gentle, classic charm, but with a lingering warmth and underlying spiciness that are entirely modern.

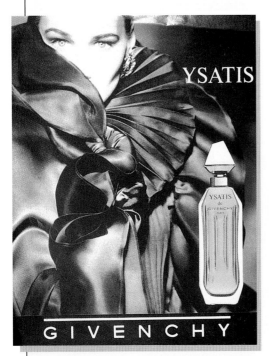

Left: Givenchy described Ysatis as a 'rendezvous between seductive charm and perfume', tailored for 'a woman of a thousand contrasting moods...refined, sophisticated, elegant'.

EXTRAVAGANCE D'AMARIGE

Launch: 1998
▲ Top notes: Green mandarin, Tagetes, Pink peppercorn, Nettle
▲ Middle notes: Jasmin, Orange blossom, Wisteria, Wild strawberry, Violet leaves
▲ Base notes: Sandalwood, Cedar, Ambrox, Black iris
Style: A sister fragrance to the hugely successful *Amarige*, this is a rather more sassy floral-fruity blend with sharp, spicy undertones. Its touch of eccentricity and daring in keeping with the new Givenchy style is reflected in the advertising, where Eva Herzigova — wearing an immaculate decollet gown designed by Alexander McQueen — sports a tattoo on her left shoulder. To launch the fragrance, a copy of the tattoo, in the form of a transfer impregnated with perfume, was given free with every bottle.

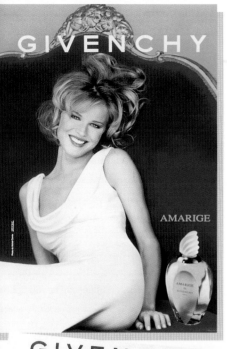

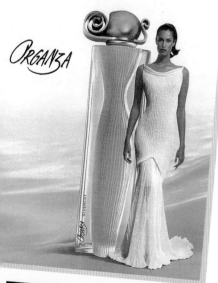

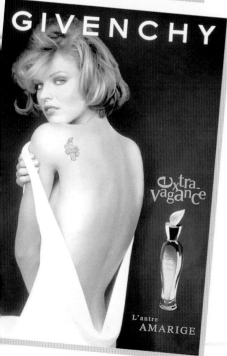

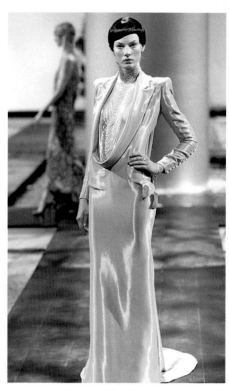

Hepburn. Two masculine perfumes, *Monsieur Givenchy* and *L'Eau de Vetyver*, followed two years later.

The 1970s and 1980s saw Givenchy tune into the new mood of independence and freedom. An exhilarating chypre-style perfume, *Givenchy III*, was created for the modern woman. *Eau de Givenchy* exudes vitality and *joie de vivre*, and *Ysatis*, packaged in a prize-winning bottle by Pierre Dinand, was a huge and instant success. A further cluster of wonderful new fragrances followed in the 1990s, among them the radiant *Amarige* and captivating *Organza*, now Givenchy's most popular perfume.

Above: This gown is from the summer 1998 show of Alexander McQueen, who became head designer at Givenchy in 1996.

PROFILE

Givenchy

1927	Hubert de Givenchy born in Beauvais, France.
1945	Goes to Paris to work for top designer Jacques Fath and study at the Ecole des Beaux Arts.
1947	Joins Elsa Schiaparelli.
1952	Opens House of Givenchy; presents first collection in Paris.
1953	Meets Balenciaga and Audrey Hepburn.
1955	Receives costume design Oscar for *Sabrina*.
1957	Founds Parfums Givenchy; launches *Le de Givenchy* and *L'Interdit*.
1959	Launches first masculine fragrance, *Monsieur de Givenchy*.
1986	Parfums Givenchy becomes part of Louis Vuitton Moët Chandon.
1995	Hubert de Givenchy retires.
1996	John Galliano appointed chief designer at Givenchy; succeeded by Alexander McQueen in October.

PERFUME CHRONOLOGY

1957	*Le de Givenchy*
1957	*L'Interdit*
1970	*Givenchy III*
1980	*Eau de Givenchy*
1984	*Ysatis*
1991	*Amarige*
1994	*Fleur d'Interdit*
1996	*Organza*
1998	*Extravagance d'Amarige*

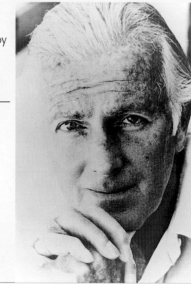

LANCÔME

The house of Lancôme was founded by a protégé of François Coty, who shared his mentor's nose for a fine fragrance and his flair for business.

The economic depression of the 1930s left the French cosmetic and perfume industries in the doldrums. American companies, such as Harriet Hubbard Ayer and Elizabeth Arden, leapt eagerly into the breach, distributing and making their 'modern' products in Europe

Right and below: Armand Petitjean was a celebrated 'nose' at Coty, and lost no time in creating new fragrances for Lancôme. Tropiques (left) was his personal favourite among the first batch launched in 1935.

and marketing them aggressively. Armand Petitjean, former director of Coty, founded Lancôme in 1935 to restore French perfumery to what he felt was its rightful supremacy.

The new company, named after a chateau in Touraine, was launched with a flourish of no fewer than five perfumes – *Tropiques*, *Kypré*, *Tendres Nuits*, *Bocages* and *Conquête*. Petitjean felt that if couturiers could launch design collections, so too could perfumers.

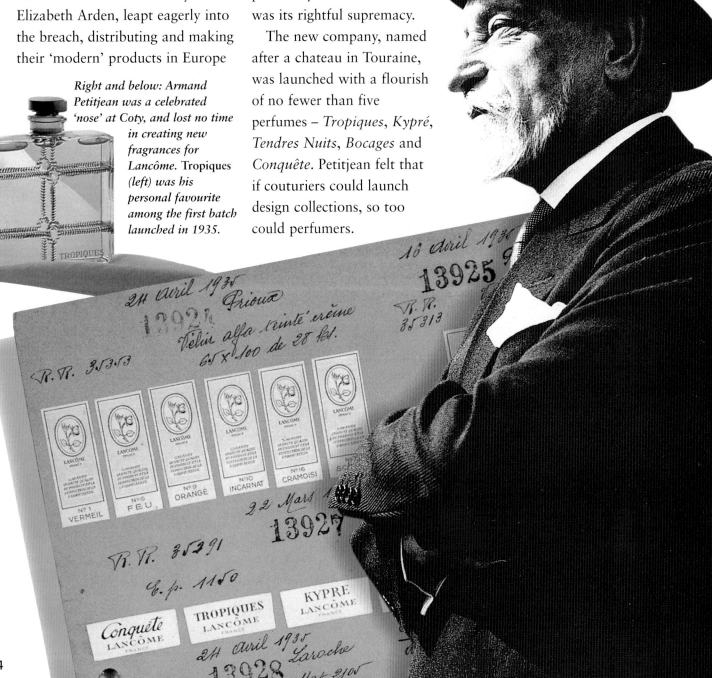

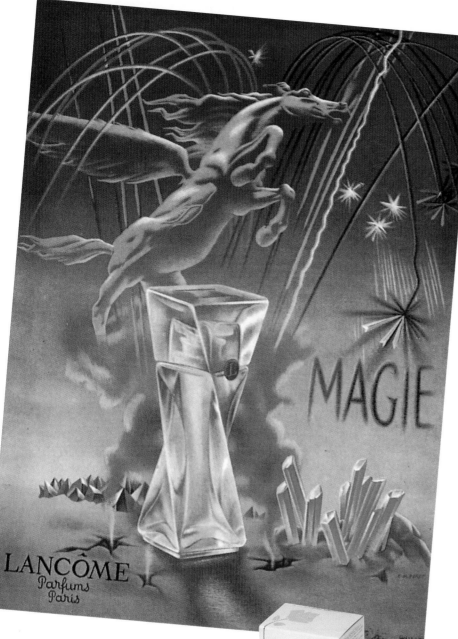

LANCÔME
*Parfums
Paris*

appeared two at a time: *Magie* was followed in 1952 by *Trésor* and *Plaisir*, then in 1957 by *Flèches d'Or* and *Envol*. The launches were lavish affairs. The one for *Trésor* in the Palais de Chaillot involved a specially commissioned ballet. Lancôme now had over 500 employees. However, Petitjean over-reached himself by building an expensive factory outside Paris and, by the end of the 1950s, the company was in financial difficulties.

CHANGE OF OWNERSHIP
Petitjean retired in 1963 and the French cosmetics giant L'Oréal took over, allowing Lancôme to take advantage of L'Oréal's state-of-the-art research laboratories. From the start, cosmetics and skin-care products had been as important to Lancôme as perfume. In 1936, they introduced a new product, *Nutrix*, a revolutionary serum-based night cream. It

Like his mentor, François Coty, Petitjean appreciated the role played by packaging in the success of a perfume. The painter Georges Delhomme, also ex-Coty, was artistic director of the new company for almost 30 years, creating some of the most intensely romantic and inventive images in perfume and designing the bottles for most Lancôme fragrances.

The 1950s were a heady time for Lancôme. New perfumes

Above: The success of Magie *in 1950 had much to do with its bottle, designed by Delhomme and manufactured by Baccarat.*

Right: Isabella Rossellini, the daughter of Ingrid Bergman and Roberto Rossellini, was the 'face' of Lancôme for 14 years, giving the company a new, more adventurous image.

Above: The Lancôme range has always included cosmetics and skin-care products, as well as fragrances.

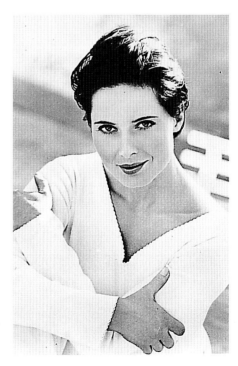

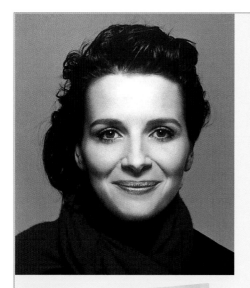

Lancôme

1935	Founded by Armand Petitjean. Five perfumes launched.
1936	Launch of *Nutrix* night cream.
1946	Lancôme introduced to the UK.
1950	Launch of worldwide bestseller perfume *Magie*.
1963	Petitjean retires.
1964	Launch of the original *Trésor* – first perfume not created by Petitjean.
1964	Company taken over by L'Oréal.
1983	Begins 14-year association with Isabella Rossellini.
1990	New *Trésor* launched to worldwide acclaim.
1996	New 'faces' of Lancôme include Juliette Binoche (left) and Marie Gillain.

PERFUME CHRONOLOGY

1935	Conquête	**1945**	Lavandes	**1969**	Ô de Lancôme
1935	Bocages	**1946**	Marrakech	**1971**	Sikkim
1935	Kypré	**1950**	Magie	**1978**	Magie Noire
1935	Tropiques	**1952**	Trésor (original)	**1990**	Trésor (new)
1935	Tendres Nuits	**1952**	Plaisir	**1995**	Poême
1937	Gardenia	**1967**	Climat	**1998**	Ô Oui!

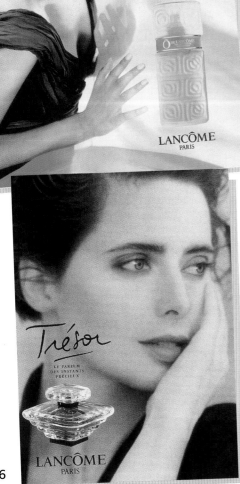

Left: Although a unisex fragrance, Ô de Lancôme's lovely freshness is particularly appealing to women.

Below left: The success of Trésor in 1990 was boosted by advertising featuring its inspiration, Isabella Rossellini.

Lancôme
COLLECTION

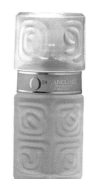

Ô DE LANCÔME

Launch date: 1969
- ▲ Top notes: Mandarin, Lemon, Bergamot, Honeysuckle, Jasmin, Grapefruit, Water lily
- ▲ Middle notes: Rosemary, Basil, Coriander
- ▲ Base notes: Oakmoss, Witchhazel

Style: This clean, refreshing foug re fragrance with citrus notes and gentle herbal undertones was conceived as a unisex scent in *eau fra che* and *eau de toilette* strengths, innovative in 1969. It was reformulated in 1995 with added ingredients.

TRÉSOR

Launch date: 1990
- ▲ Top notes: White rose, Apricot blossom, Lily-of-the-valley
- ▲ Middle notes: Iris, Heliotrope, Lilac
- ▲ Base notes: Peach, Vanilla, Sandalwood, Amber, Musk

Style: *Tr sor* was created by Russian-American perfumer Sophia Grojsman, who called it a warm, hug me fragrance. The heady scents of fresh flowers mingle with soft powdery fruits and spicy woods in an intensely feminine modern classic inspired by the Face of Lanc me, Isabella Rossellini.

The bottle is an upside-down pyramid, designed by Areca to be held in the palm of the hand. It carries the same name as the hugely successful Lanc me perfume of 1952.

established the Lancôme reputation for innovative skin treatments and cosmetics. In the 1960s they anticipated the new 'no-make-up' look with soft brown and beige eyeshadow palettes, and in the 1980s they revolutionized the marketing of make-up with spring and autumn collections in fashionable colour ranges.

THE FACE OF LANCÔME

The first autumn collection was the début of Isabella Rossellini as the 'face' of Lancôme, a position that

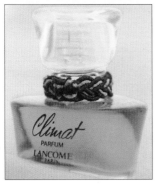

Left: Climat *was the first successful fragrance launched by Lancôme after it was taken over by L'Oréal in the 1960s.*

she would hold for 14 years. The new version of *Trésor*, launched in 1990, was the fragrance most closely linked with her. Lancôme's first new perfume for 12 years, it was dazzlingly successful, and soon became the world's leading fragrance. This triumph was followed by the flowery oriental *Poême*

and then by *Ô Oui!*, which was a complete contrast. Unashamedly youthful, joyous and optimistic, *Ô Oui!* is designed to take the Lancôme fragrance repertoire forward into a new century with a new mood for a new generation.

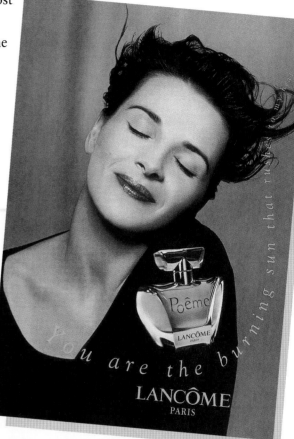

P O Ê M E

Launch date: 1995

▲ Notes: Himalayan blue poppy, Datura, Mimosa, Jonquil, Freesia, Rose, Jasmin, Daffodil, Vanilla flowers

Style: Composed entirely of florals by master perfumer Jacques Cavallier — who abandoned the traditional structure of top, middle and base notes — *Po me* is an irresistible blend of exotic blooms and fresh spring flowers. This dynamic contrast of opposites resolves into a close rhythmic harmony that is both classic and contemporary. The bottle was described by its creator, Fabien Baron, as a prism that transfigures light as poetry transforms reality .

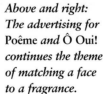

Above and right: The advertising for Poême *and* Ô Oui! *continues the theme of matching a face to a fragrance.*

Ô O U I !

Launch date: 1998

▲ Top notes: Bergamot, Clementine, Water hyacinth, Nectarine, Freesia

▲ Middle notes: Pear, Pineapple, Honeysuckle, Stephanotis

▲ Base note: Stargazer lily

Style: Exuding fresh, youthful vitality and *joie de vivre,* this bright, clean, wide-awake *eau fra che* has sharp, citrus top notes that blend easily with sweet fruits and the lingering warmth of lilies. The perfume, aimed at the youth market and with a name signifying Say yes to life! , has a silver-topped frosted bottle similar to that of de Lanc me and was designed by Serge Mansau.

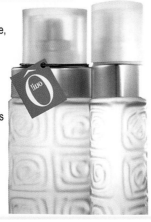

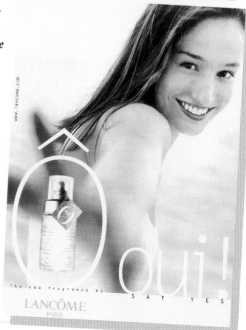

GUERLAIN

One of France's oldest perfume houses, Guerlain has maintained a centuries-old tradition of creating fragrances to capture the spirit of the age.

The young Jean-Paul Guerlain took over the perfumer's chair at the House of Guerlain in 1956. He was heir to a company that had grown from a tiny shop in Paris to a huge international business, and a family tradition over a century old.

Three previous generations of Guerlains had created nearly 300 fragrances, including such stars as *Eau Imperiale*, *Jicky*, *L'Heure Bleue*, *Mitsouko*, *Vol de Nuit* and *Shalimar*. Each generation had made perfumes to match the spirit of the age. It was Jean-Paul's task to do the same for the modern world.

GREAT GIFT

Fortunately, he was very talented. His gift had been spotted by his grandfather, Jacques, who coached him from an early age, training him to hone his olfactory memory. At 18, he collaborated with Jacques to create *Ode*, his first perfume and his grandfather's last. The first fragrance he created on his own was for men. *Vétiver* was inspired by a family

Far left: Guerlain's Beauty Institute on the Champs-Elysées is considered a national monument.
Left: Vétiver, Jean-Paul Guerlain's first solo creation, was released in 1959.

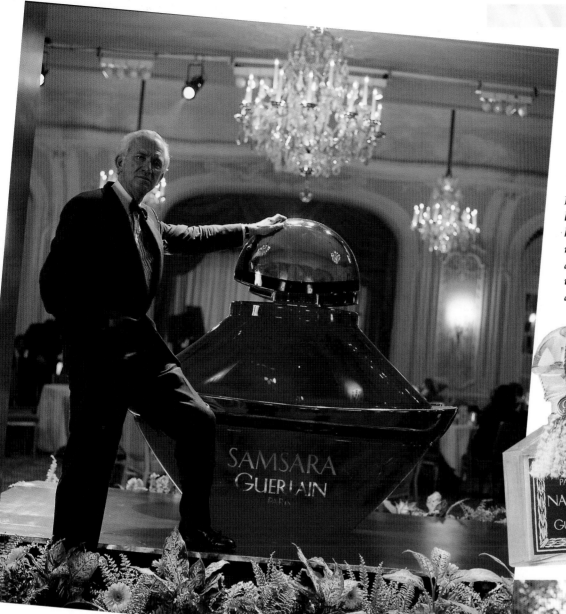

Below: Nahéma, launched in 1979, has top notes of roses and peaches and a base of woody notes and vanilla.

gardener, who smelled comfortably of earth and grass mingled with tobacco.

Like most creative people, Jean-Paul needed a muse, and for many of his female fragrances he had a particular woman in mind. For *Chant d'Arômes* (1962), it was an early love; for *Chamade* (1969), a mysterious but 'very, very beautiful' woman; for *Parure* (1975), it was his mother; and for *Nahéma* (1979), Catherine Deneuve. *Samsara* (1989), a heady blend of sandalwood and jasmin, was created to seduce an elegant Englishwoman, who wore it for four years before its launch.

Above: Samsara *marked the first time that Guerlain had created a perfume to fit a preconceived idea, rather than finding a concept that described a new fragrance.*

Right: Catherine Deneuve starred in La Chamade, *a film based on the Françoise Sagan novel that gave Guerlain the name for his perfume. The actress herself inspired Guerlain to create* Nahéma.

In the 1970s and '80s, there was intense competition among proliferating company names and fragrances, and many perfume houses sold out to large conglomerates in order to survive. However, Guerlain, like Chanel and Patou, continued to develop and produce their own perfumes. The family tradition was never to compromise on quality. Synthetics were only used as complements to expensive natural substances, never as substitutes for them.

NEW SCENTS FOR A NEW AGE

In the late 1980s, in a reaction against the materialism and stress of the modern world, people began to seek more spiritual values in Eastern religions. Guerlain wanted to produce a perfume to evoke this mood. After numerous trials, the classic oriental mix of jasmin and sandalwood proved the answer. It was christened *Samsara* – a Sanskrit word meaning 'eternal return' and symbolizing the cycle of life, death and rebirth. It was then packaged in a bottle, whose shape was inspired by an old Cambodian temple sculpture seen in a Paris museum. Launched in 1989, exactly 100 years after the great *Jicky*, under the slogan 'the search for serenity', *Samsara* marked Guerlain's final confident adjustment to the modern world. It is now the company's best-selling fragrance.

The ability to adapt to new conditions has enabled Guerlain to maintain its identity. Although it is now owned by Louis Vuitton-Moët-Hennessey, the company is still run and controlled by the Guerlain family, and the vital traditions of creativity and excellence transmitted from one generation to the next still survive.

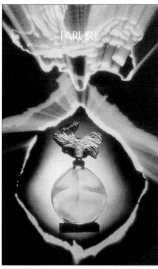

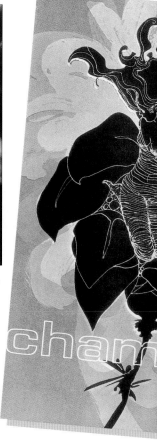

Above and right: Striking advertisements, in the graphic style of the time, have always been used to promote Guerlain scents.

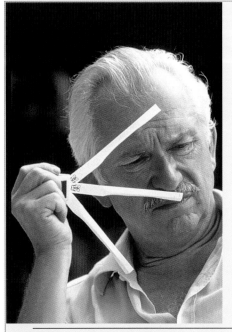

Guerlain

PROFILE

1955	Launch of *Ode*, Jacques Guerlain's last perfume and Jean-Paul's first.
1956	Jacques retires; Jean-Paul (left) becomes the new 'nose'.
1964	Philippe Guerlain takes over the running of the company.
1970	Bottle designer Raymond Guerlain dies; is succeeded by Robert Granai.
1973	New manufacturing plant built at Chartres.
1973	Subsidiaries opened in Hong Kong and Tokyo.
1980	Launch of Issima skincare line.
1986	New boutique opens on Boulevard Haussman, Paris.
1989	Sixth shop opens in Montparnasse in Paris.
1991	L'Or de Guerlain cosmetics launched.
1992	Seventh shop opens on Rue Bonaparte in Paris.
1993	Beauty Institute is revamped.
1994	Launch of *Petit Guerlain*, the company's first scent for children.
1996	Lavish Beauty Institute and exclusive boutique opens in Toulouse; launch of Perfect Light cosmetic line.

PERFUME CHRONOLOGY

1955	*Ode*	**1969**	*Chamade*	**1979**	*Nahéma*	**1994**	*Petit Guerlain (for children)*
1959	*Vétiver (for men)*	**1974**	*Eau de Guerlain*	**1983**	*Jardins de Bagatelle*		
1962	*Chant d'Arômes*	**1975**	*Parure*	**1989**	*Samsara*	**1995**	*un Air de Samsara*
1965	*Habit Rouge (for men)*	**1978**	*Silences*	**1992**	*Héritage (for men)*	**1996**	*Champs-Elysées*

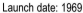

Guerlain
COLLECTION

CHAMADE

Launch date: 1969

▲ Top notes: Hyacinth, Galbanum

▲ Middle notes: Ylang-ylang, Blackcurrant bud, Rose, Jasmin
(Hedione, synthetic jasmin fragrance)

▲ Base notes: Vanilla, Woods, Iris, Tonka bean

Style: The first of Jean-Paul Guerlain s great feminine perfumes is intensely seductive and sensual. A bouquet of sweet-smelling flowers is refreshed by hyacinth and warmed by fruity blackcurrant buds — the first time this ingredient had been used in a perfume. Some say the bottle, designed by Raymond Guerlain, is a stylized shell; others that it is a heart turned over in response to the chamade , a military drum roll that signals a retreat.

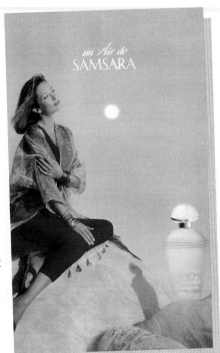

JARDINS DE BAGATELLE

Launch date: 1983

▲ Top note: Violet, Lemon, Bergamot

▲ Neroli, Rose, Jasmin, Gardenia, Magnolia, Tuberose

▲ Base notes: Cedarwood, V tiver, Patchouli

Style: This is a radiant, open-air perfume, full of bright spontaneity and joy, in which the delicate fragrance of mixed white blossom is heightened by the intoxicating scent of tuberose. It is named after the famous rose gardens in the Bois de Boulogne, created for Marie Antoinette in 1777.

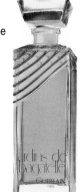

UN AIR DE SAMSARA

Launch date: 1995

▲ Top note: Bergamot, Lemon, Mint, Leafy notes

▲ Middle notes: Narcissus, Jasmin

▲ Base notes: Sandalwood

Style: Guerlain produced un Air de Samsara as a lighter, slightly fresher version of his top-selling oriental-style fragrance, Samsara. A rush of citrus and mint gives way to a fresh, floral fragrance underpinned with sandalwood from Guerlain s Indian plantations, which were bought to ensure future supplies for Samsara.

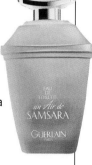

CHAMPS ELYSÉES

Launch date: 1996

▲ Top notes: Rose petal, Mimosa leaf, Almond blossom

▲ Middle notes: Mimosa blossom, Buddleia

▲ Base notes: Hibiscus seed, Almond wood

Style: This fresh, natural fragrance with a hint of boldness symbolizes the modern liberated woman. It mixes light, delicate florals with the warm, mildly exotic accents of mimosa, almond wood and hibiscus to exude a gentle confidence and a bright, happy accord. The angular bottle echoes architectural features in and around the Champs-Elys es in Paris.

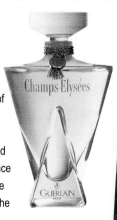

Left and right: The advertising for **Jardins de Bagatelle** *and* **Champs-Elysées** *expresses their distinct styles – the one floral and joyous, the other assured and liberated.*

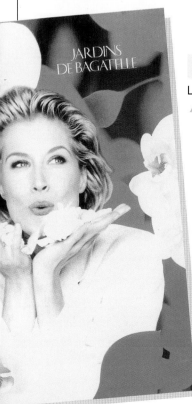

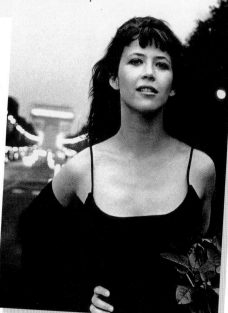

JEAN PAUL GAULTIER

Although he is famous as the lovable bad boy or clown prince of French fashion, Jean Paul Gaultier is a highly skilled designer and cultural innovator.

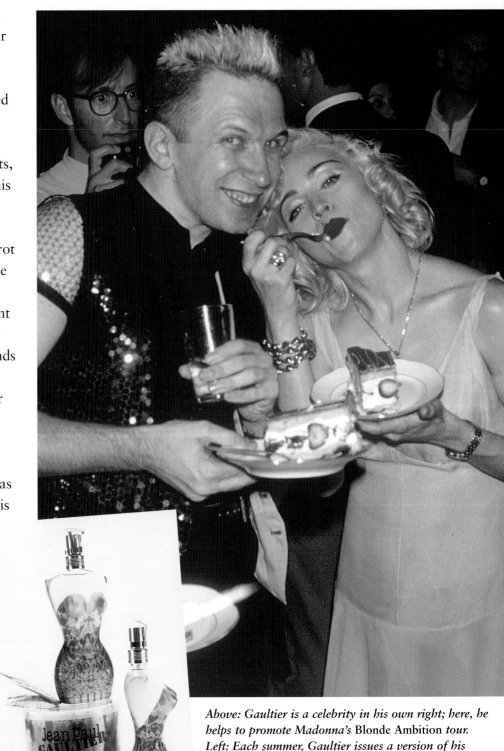

The man who had women wear corsets in the street, put men in tutus and sent Madonna on a world tour in a pink satin pointed bra was born in the suburbs of Paris in 1952. The only child of two loving, if distant, accountants, he spent much of his time with his richly eccentric grandmother.

She was the main influence in his life and work. Variously a tarot reader, palmist, faith healer, nurse and beautician, she not only recognized and nurtured his talent but also provided a rich seam of indelible memories of sights, sounds and smells that he would later plunder repeatedly for ideas. Her wonderfully elaborate 1950s' undergarments inspired his 'underwear as outerwear' revolution, for example, as well as the curvaceous body bottle for his first female fragrance.

FAMOUS FACE

Gaultier's giggly appearances on *Eurotrash* have made him instantly recognizable far beyond the rarefied confines of the fashion world. His faintly comical looks – big and beefy, with bleached, cropped hair, wearing a striped *matelot* T-shirt, kilt and Doc Martens

Above: Gaultier is a celebrity in his own right; here, he helps to promote Madonna's Blonde Ambition *tour. Left: Each summer, Gaultier issues a version of his fragrance with a new dress for its body bottle.*

boots – are worlds away from the urbane image of the French couturier, yet it was Pierre Cardin who gave him his first break, aged 17, and who provided his vital grounding in cutting and tailoring.

After brief stints with Esterel and Patou, he finally gathered the confidence to break out on his own. With a loan from a friend, he launched his first ready-to-wear collection in 1976 in the Palais de la Découverte, a former music hall. The models wore biker jackets and 'table-mat' dresses made of straw. Only 16 people came.

LONG STRUGGLE

The next few years were a struggle to survive, but he persisted with a bubbling torrent of designs drawn from a wildly eclectic mix of stylistic references – street fashion, the 1950s, ethnic clothes, fetishes, tattoos and piercings, fairy tales and the movies. He loved Brando in *The Wild One* and the glamour of 1950s' sweater girls, such as Lana Turner and Ava Gardner.

Television appearances, records and costume designs for cult films made Gaultier as much a star as any of his clients. He launched two new clothing lines, Junior Gaultier and Gaultier Jeans, and, in 1993, his first perfume for women.

For its inspiration, he returned to his remarkable grandmother – the sweet, powdery smell of make-up in her bedroom, and the theatre she took him to as a child, the sharp resinous odour of nail polish and the scent of flowers in her room.

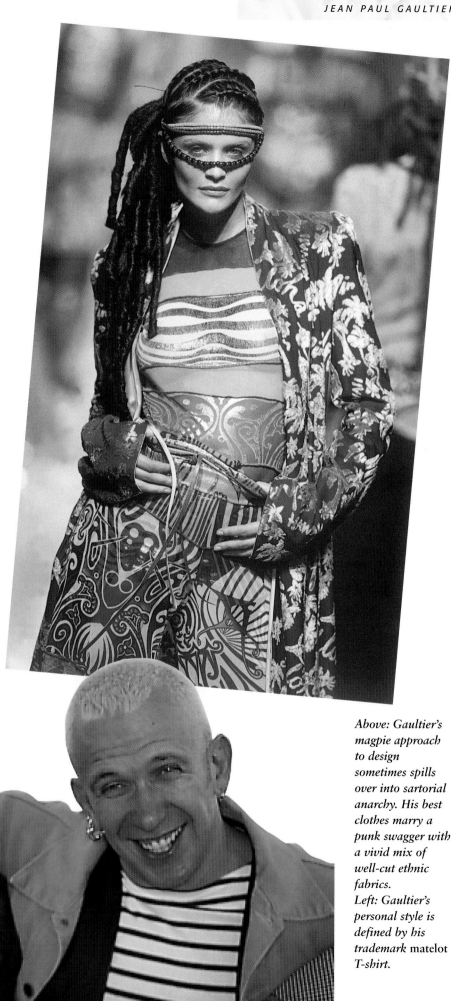

Above: Gaultier's magpie approach to design sometimes spills over into sartorial anarchy. His best clothes marry a punk swagger with a vivid mix of well-cut ethnic fabrics.
Left: Gaultier's personal style is defined by his trademark matelot *T-shirt.*

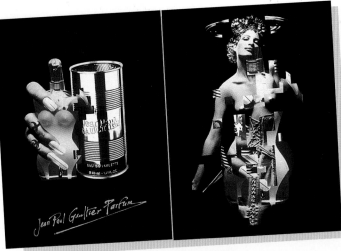

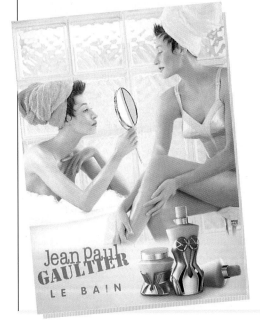

Above and below: Gaultier's advertising for both his perfume and bath range is as quirky and inventive as the products themselves.

Jean Paul Gaultier
COLLECTION

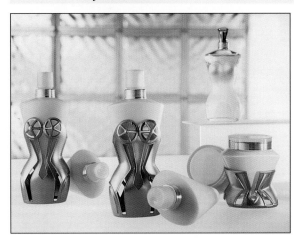

JEAN PAUL GAULTIER

Launch: 1993

▲ Top notes: Orange blossom, Rose, Mandarin, Star anise
▲ Middle notes: Orchid, Florentine orris, Ylang-ylang, Ginger
▲ Base notes: Vanilla, Amber

Style: This is an ultra-feminine, almost old-fashioned fragrance with soft, flowery top notes, a silky, spicy heart and warm, woody base. For the extrait , the flesh-pink corset bottle is encased in copper fretwork lacing, while the eau de toilette refillable spray has a coppery sheath dress. All are encased in silver tin can packages that hark back to one of Gaultier s early jewellery experiments, when he made bangles out of cans.

JEAN PAUL GAULTIER LE BAIN

This complementary range of toiletries, in packaging that echoes the pink body bottle, comprises a bath and shower gel, body lotion and body cream to cleanse, moisturize and nourish the skin. They include honey derivatives, hibiscus and orchid extracts and ceramides to help protect and balance the skin s natural oils.

The pink body bottle with its frosted corset was not, as some said, a copy of Schiaparelli's famous flaçon for *Shocking*, but another homage to grandmother's lingerie. The bottle for his men's fragrance, *Le Male*, pays tribute to another Gaultier signature, the *matelot* T-shirt, clinging to an overtly male torso. Inside the bottle, though, is a traditional lavender water.

By the late 1990s, Gaultier had matured not only in years, but in experience and creative ambition.

In 1996 he produced his first *haute couture* collection. Dior made a tentative approach, and there was a definite offer from Givenchy but, typically, he preferred independence.

Today, the doyennes of the fashion world fight to attend his couture shows; they have become extravaganzas of showbiz spectacle and magnificently assured – but still startlingly original – clothes.

Right: By the time of his autumn-spring collection of 1996–97, Gaultier's style was moving towards haute couture.

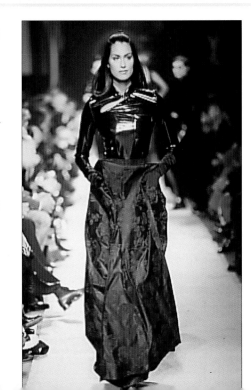

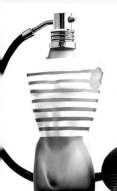

LE MALE

Launch: 1995

▲ Top notes: Artemisia, Spearmint, Bergamot, Cardamom
▲ Middle notes: Lavender, Orange blossom, Cinnamon, Cumin
▲ Base notes: Cedar, Sandalwood, Musk, Amber, Vanilla, Tonka bean
Style: A revamped classic — typically, Gaultier has reworked the masculine tradition of lavender water — this eau de toilette has sharp, lemony top notes and an oriental-style, fleshy, warm base. The prestige version of the scent revives another tradition; the male torso bottle is crowned with a silk-tasselled, rubber-bulbed spray, like those on toilet waters in an old-time barber s shop.

LE MALE RANGE

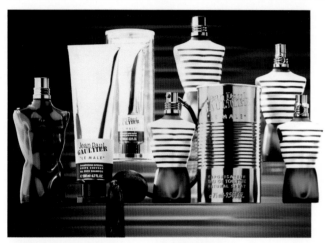

The after-shave lotion includes witch hazel softened with aloe vera to soothe razor burn, and is scented with bursts of mint and lavender. The alcohol-free after-shave gel, sold in a tube like toothpaste, has wheatgrain extract added to the lotion ingredients. The all-over honey-enriched shower shampoo is a gentle foam that soothes and moisturizes the skin and makes hair clean and shiny.

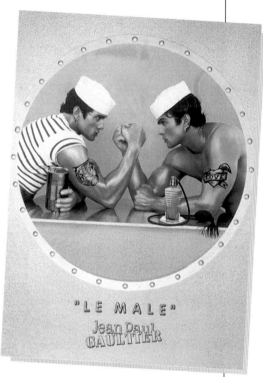

"LE MALE"
Jean Paul GAULTIER

Above: The camp advertising for Le Male is typical of the way Gaultier uses his outrageous image to work in his favour.

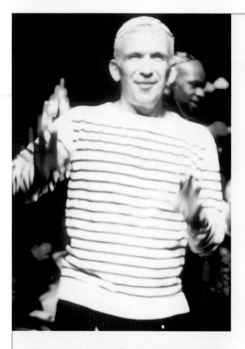

PERFUME CHRONOLOGY

1993 *Jean Paul Gaultier*
1995 *Le Male*

Jean Paul Gaultier

1952 Jean Paul Gaultier born 24 April in Arcueil, Paris.
1970 Joins Pierre Cardin as design assistant.
1974 Appointed designer for Cardin US Collection, working in the Philippines.
1976 Launches first ready-to-wear collection under his own name.
1985 Introduces skirts for men in the 'And God Created Man' collection.
1987 Wins Fashion Oscar Award in Paris.
1988 'Le Concierge' women's collection – underwear as outerwear. Starts Junior Gaultier with Fiorucci.
1989 Designs costumes for Helen Mirren in Peter Greenaway's *The Thief, The Cook, His Wife and Her Lover*.
1990 Designs costumes for Madonna's *Blonde Ambition* world tour.
1991 First combined male-female collection 'Adam et Eve Rastas d' Aujourd'hui'.
1992 Starts Gaultier Jeans; mounts star-studded retrospective in Los Angeles in aid of HIV research.
1993 Launches first women's perfume *Jean Paul Gaultier*.
1993 First appearance on *Eurotrash*.
1994 Designs costumes for Victoria Abril in Pedro Almodovar's *Kika*. Launch of JPG budget line to replace Junior Gaultier.
1995 First men's fragrance *Le Male*.
1996 First couture show.

ELIZABETH ARDEN

Her strong will, boundless confidence and marketing flair helped Elizabeth Arden build a beauty-care business into one of the great American perfume houses.

prepare ointments and medicines. She soon decided to abandon her nursing career and open her own beauty salon, using recipes from her chemist friend.

BEHIND THE RED DOOR

New York was the obvious place to start. There were more wealthy, sophisticated women there. She worked for the beautician Eleanor Adair to gain experience, then left in 1910 to open her own shop on Fifth Avenue. The entire place was

Left: Elizabeth Arden was a tyrannical employer given to sudden rages, but was also a creative, energetic businesswoman. Below: Blue Grass, *her first perfume, was named in honour of her home in Virginia.*

Elizabeth Arden was born Florence Nightingale Graham near Toronto in 1878, the daughter of poor English-Scots immigrants. True to her name, she enrolled on a nursing course, but the sight of blood horrified her and she sought refuge from the wards of the Toronto hospital in the laboratories, where she helped the chemist

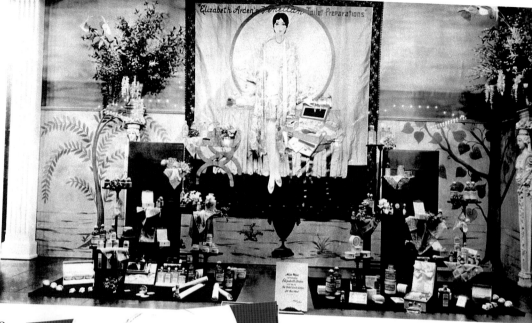

Right: In the early years, Elizabeth Arden was renowned for her beauty products. This display shows the Venetian range.

decorated in damask pink, except for the door, which was painted a bright lacquer red. She adopted the name Elizabeth Arden, and the bright red door became her signature.

Soldiers returning from France after World War I had brought back all kinds of cosmetics and perfumes, which did much to soften the puritanical attitudes of American women to beauty products. This was good news for the beauty business.

The Arden empire flourished, driven by Elizabeth's ambition and her fierce competitiveness, especially with her life-long rival, Helena Rubinstein. Salons were opened in Paris and London, as well as the USA, and the beauty products were also sold in department stores. By 1925 the company was grossing $20 million

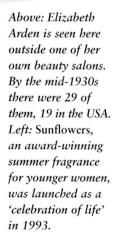

a year; five years later, it made $80 million, with 108 different beauty products on the market.

FIRST FRAGRANCES

Arden first moved into the perfume business by buying the US rights to Babani of Paris, and in 1935 launched *Blue Grass*, one of the world's classic floral-oriental fragrances, created by the Grasse perfumers Roure. It remained a world best-seller for several decades.

It was followed by others, including *Cyclamen*, *It's You* and *On Dit*. Like all Arden fragrances, they were made by French perfumers. The bottle for *Cyclamen*, designed by Baccarat, included a detachable floral pin that could be worn as jewellery.

The company continued to open salons all over the world, with the same pink interior and bright red door. Elizabeth Arden herself worked ceaselessly until her death

Above: Elizabeth Arden is seen here outside one of her own beauty salons. By the mid-1930s there were 29 of them, 19 in the USA. Left: Sunflowers, an award-winning summer fragrance for younger women, was launched as a 'celebration of life' in 1993.

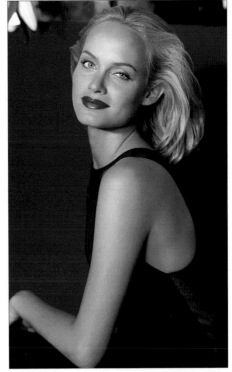

Right: Amber Valletta is the current 'face' of Elizabeth Arden, featuring in the launch of the new fragrance, Splendor.

in 1966. She was 87, but looked 60, had the energy of someone half her age and, until then, had seemed indestructible. She left the company to relatives, who sold out to a pharmaceutical company. The Simply Perfect make-up range, launched in 1986, was a sensational success, introducing Elizabeth Arden to younger women.

NEW VENTURES

Following links with Lagerfeld, Valentino, Fendi, Cerruti, Elizabeth Taylor and Fabergé, the Elizabeth Arden company passed to Unilever in 1989, but still honours the memory of its extraordinary creator; the launch of the perfume *Red Door* in 1989 commemorated her famous informal trademark.

PROFILE

Elizabeth Arden

1878	Born Florence Nightingale Graham on 31 December near Toronto, Canada.
1908	Begins work as beauty treatment assistant for Eleanor Adair in New York.
1910	Opens own beauty salon on Fifth Avenue as Elizabeth Arden.
1920	Opens first European salon in Rue St Honoré, Paris, managed by her sister Gladys, and another in Old Bond Street, London.
1930	Opens purpose-built factory in West London.
1932	Introduces her first Colour Harmony lipstick 'wardrobe'.
1934	Opens her home, Maine Chance, as a beauty and health retreat.
1935	Launches first perfume *Blue Grass*.
1953	Launches line of men's toiletries.
1966	Elizabeth Arden dies on 21 October.
1987	Company bought by Fabergé.
1989	Company bought by Unilever.
1994	Elizabeth Arden's Red Door salon re-opens in London in Simpsons, Piccadilly.

PERFUME CHRONOLOGY

1935	*Blue Grass*	**1989**	*Blue Grass*
1938	*Cyclamen*		relaunch
1939	*It's You*	**1993**	*Sunflowers*
1944	*On Dit*	**1995**	*True Love*
1957	*Mémoire; Chérie*	**1996**	*5th Avenue*
1974	*Eau Fraîche*	**1996**	*Red Door*
1977	*Cabriole*		relaunch
1989	*Red Door*	**1999**	*Splendor*

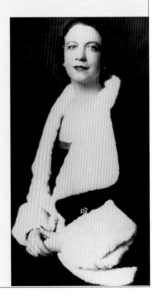

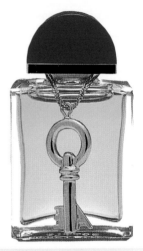

Elizabeth Arden
COLLECTION

RED DOOR

Launch: 1989

▲ Top notes: Rose, Ylang-ylang

▲ Middle notes: Jasmin, Lily-of-the-valley, Orchid, Orange blossom, Lily, Freesia, Violet

▲ Base notes: Vetiver, Amber, Musk, Benzoin

Style: A floral-oriental blend of sensuous flower fragrances with spicy vetiver undertones, this fragrance was named after the traditional entrance to Elizabeth Arden beauty salons. It was relaunched in 1996 with Linda Evangelista as the face.

Below: The vivid lacquer red of the stopper of **Red Door** *has long been an Arden signature colour.*

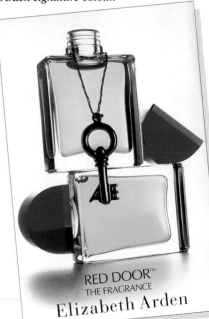

RED DOOR™
THE FRAGRANCE
Elizabeth Arden

TRUE LOVE

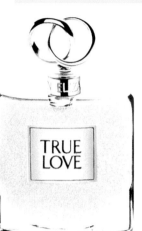

Launch: 1995
▲ Top notes: Freesia, Lily-of-the-valley, Rose
▲ Middle notes: Jasmin, Lotus, Iris, Narcissus
▲ Base notes: Sandalwood, Vetiver, Musk
Style: This markedly floral perfume, created by Alain Astori, uses a process in which the combined rose and lotus notes create a new harmony. The romantic theme of the scent and name is carried over on to the bottle; there is a gold band, like a wedding ring, around the neck, and two more interlocked on the stopper.

Right: True Love's ad deliberately promotes the traditional romantic image of love and marriage.

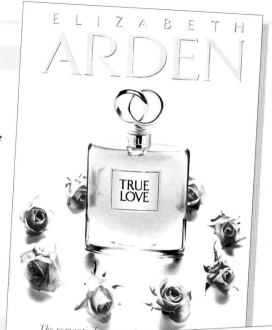

5TH AVENUE

Launch: 1996
▲ Top notes: Lilac, Linden, Magnolia, Lily-of-the-valley, Mandarin, Bergamot
▲ Middle notes: Rose, Violet, Ylang-ylang, Jasmin, Tuberose
▲ Base notes: Amber, Musk, Sandalwood, Orris, Vanilla
Style: In a streamlined bottle inspired by the Manhattan skyline, this modern American classic epitomizes the chic confidence of Fifth Avenue, New York s premier fashion street, and the home of Elizabeth Arden s first salon. It is an elegant blend of sweet floral scents woven with exotic tuberose, ylang-ylang, warm, rich spices and precious woods.

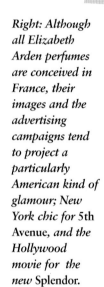

Right: Although all Elizabeth Arden perfumes are conceived in France, their images and the advertising campaigns tend to project a particularly American kind of glamour; New York chic for 5th Avenue, and the Hollywood movie for the new Splendor.

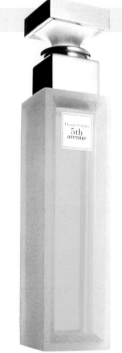

SPLENDOR

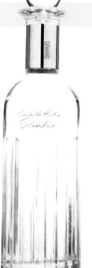

Launch: 1999
▲ Top notes: Sweet pea, Wisteria, Hyacinth, White peony, Freesia
▲ Middle notes: Water-lily, Jasmin, Magnolia, Rose, Poppy
▲ Base notes: Satinwood, Musk
Style: An exquisitely seductive floral fragrance evoking femininity and romantic joy, *Splendor* is a complex mingling of sharp intensity and softness, of the cool sweetness of water-lily and magnolia with the warmth of musk. It is packaged in a delicately fluted bottle, with a silver collar inspired by those on crystal decanters.

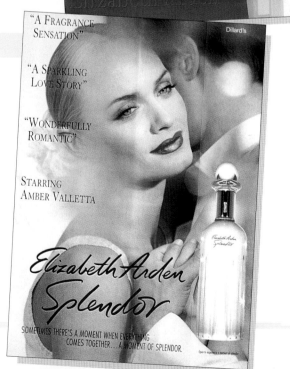

"A FRAGRANCE SENSATION"

"A SPARKLING LOVE STORY"

"WONDERFULLY ROMANTIC"

STARRING AMBER VALLETTA

Elizabeth Arden Splendor

SOMETIMES THERE'S A MOMENT WHEN EVERYTHING COMES TOGETHER...A MOMENT OF SPLENDOR.

GIANNI VERSACE

The clothes designed by Gianni Versace are the epitome of glitz and glamour, and the theme is echoed in some dazzling perfumes.

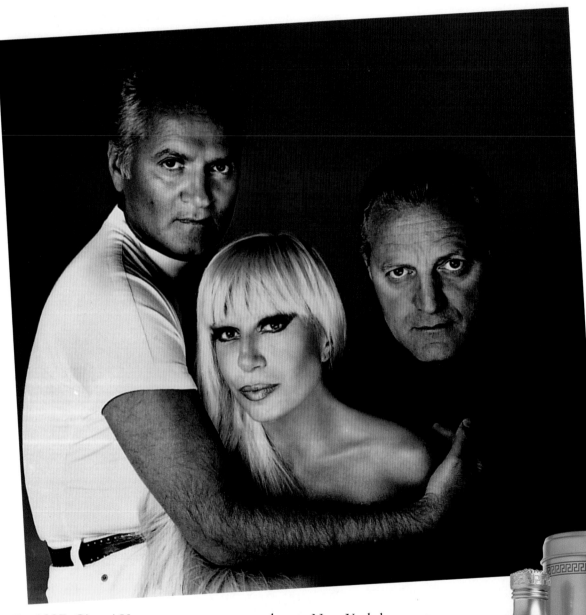

Left: Gianni Versace (far left) never forgot his family and roots. Santo, his older brother, and their sister, Donatella, were important parts of the organization from the beginning.

Below: The Jeans range, with its novel packaging, was launched to appeal to the youth market.

In 1997, Gianni Versace was living like a Renaissance prince. Fabulously wealthy, he was the jet-set's favourite designer and was showered with critical accolades. Much of his wealth was spent on art and antiques to furnish his luxurious showpiece homes: a palazzo overlooking Lake Como, an elegant New York brownstone and a glorious Mediterranean-style villa on Miami's South Beach.

In July of that year, he was gunned down outside the villa, part of a killing spree by a gay prostitute who later committed suicide. This crime brought a tragic end to a meteoric and glittering career.

Versace was born in Calabria, southern Italy, in 1946. His mother gave him his first taste of fashion, in the shape of a boutique where she made up dresses for rich

masochism. More than any other designer, he was responsible for the sharp-shouldered power-dressing of the 1980s' dominatrix.

Above all, Versace's clothes, full of visual bravado and opulent self-

confidence, attracted attention. 'I like to dress egos,' he once said, and his clients included Madonna, Demi Moore, Joan Collins, Liz Taylor, Sylvester Stallone, Elton John, Eric Clapton and Princess Diana. Actress Liz Hurley had her career made by the Versace dress that she wore to the première of *Four Weddings and a Funeral*. The next day she was on every front page, and so was Versace.

Versace knew the value of publicity and hype. His theatrical projects, designing opera and ballet costumes, and his collaboration with

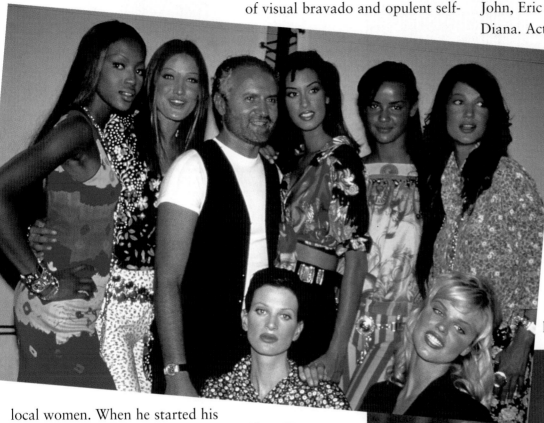

local women. When he started his own business in Milan, he brought his family with him. His brother, Santo, became his manager, while his sister, Donatella, remained his close creative partner and became chief designer after his death.

From the start, his trademark was uncompromising glitz and glamour, and an overt sexuality teetering on the edge of vulgarity.

Versace loved dramatic sculptural shapes, fetish fabrics (silk, satin, leather, rubber, chain-mail) and flamboyant colours and decoration. His eclectic sources of inspiration took in the classic designs of Poiret and Vionnet, street fashion, punk, military uniforms, ethnic costumes and, in his 1993 collection, sado-

Above: Versace dressed his models in clothes that were full of visual bravado and opulent self-confidence.

Right: After Gianni's death, Donatella, who had been his creative partner as well as the 'face' of some of his fragrances, moved into the spotlight, creating collections of her own designs.

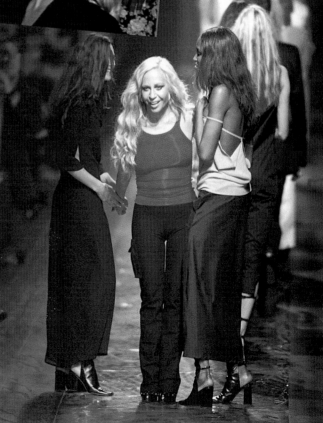

choreographer Maurice Béjart, gave him valuable creative kudos, and helped advance the idea of him as a Renaissance man.

GLAMOUR AND YOUTH

Versace launched his first fragrance, *Gianni Versace*, in 1981. This spicy, sensual, chypre-type perfume embodied his ideal woman – a strong, sexy survivor – someone, he often said, like Tina Turner. Its enormous success prompted the creation of *Versace l'Homme*, a companion fragrance for men, which was

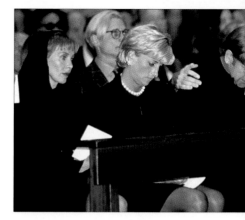

Right: Versace's position as the jet-set's favourite designer ensured a star-studded turn-out at his funeral in 1997.

launched in 1984. With its tangy top notes, heart of exotic flowers and warm, spicy base, it was aimed at sophisticated modern men. In 1988 a new division, Gianni Versace Profumi (known as 'Gi-Ver') was created to handle the perfumery.

A recurrent Versace theme is fragrances specifically designed to complement clothing lines. *Versus Donna* (1992) and *Versus Uomo* (1993) follow the Versus label, which focuses on

informal styles aimed at younger people. The *Jeans* collection of fragrances, a series of eaux de toilettes in distinctive soft-drinks-style bottles and colour-printed canisters, began in 1994. They echo the concept of Versace designer jeans; young, stylish and affordable, for those who want a touch of star-studded Versace.

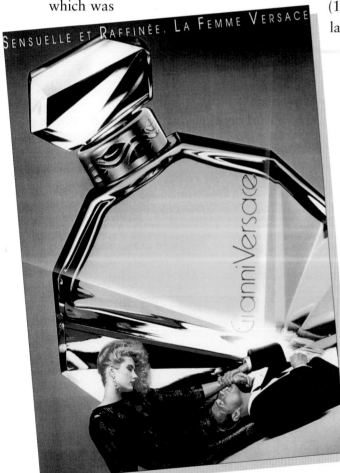

SENSUELLE ET RAFFINÉE, LA FEMME VERSACE

Above: The sculptured, asymmetric bottle was the 'star' of the launch campaign for Gianni Versace.

Versace
COLLECTION

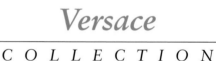

GIANNI VERSACE

Launch: 1981
▲ Top notes: Bergamot, Neroli
▲ Middle notes: Rose, Ylang-ylang, Broom, Jasmin
▲ Base notes: Sandalwood, Patchouli, Oakmoss, Tonka beans, Frankincense, Myrrh
Style: This warm, sensual, floral-chypre perfume was created by Grasse perfumers Roure, and aimed at sophisticated, yet feminine, women. Its many-faceted, sculptured bottle has a cap like a cut diamond.

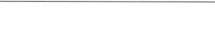

VERSUS DONNA

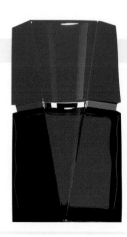

Launch: 1992
▲ Top notes: Peach, Plum, Green notes
▲ Middle notes: Rose, Tuberose, Lily-of-the-valley, Jasmin
▲ Base notes: Sandalwood, Cedar, Amber, Musk
Style: *Versus Donna* is a powdery, fruity-floral fragrance with an original structure that is based on contrasts and complementary opposites. At once vivacious and intimate, introvert and extrovert, lively and relaxing, it was designed to complement the Versus youth fashion line created in 1989.

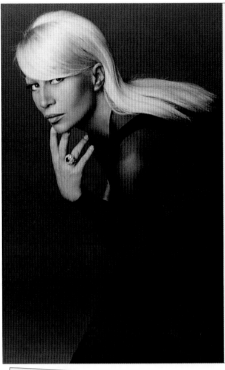

Versace

1946 Gianni Versace born in Reggio, Calabria, Italy.

1972 Presents first ready-to-wear collections for Genny and Complice in Milan.

1978 Presents first women's collection under the Versace name in Milan.

1981 Launches first women's perfume, *Gianni Versace*.

1982 Wins first of his 'L'Occhio d'Oro' awards for fashion design.

1984 Launches first men's perfume, *Versace l'Homme*.

1989 Launches the Versus line for young people.

1993 Wins the Council of Fashion Designers of America's fashion Oscar.

1997 Gianni Versace is murdered outside his home in Miami Beach. Donatella Versace (left) takes over as chief designer.

1998 Largest Versace Jeans couture shop opens in New Bond Street, London.

PERFUME CHRONOLOGY

1981 *Gianni Versace*	**1994** *Red Jeans*	**1996** *Green Jeans*
1984 *Versace l'Homme*	**1994** *Blue Jeans*	**1996** *The Dreamer*
1989 *V'E*	**1995** *Baby Rose Jeans*	**1996** *Blonde*
1992 *Versus Donna*	**1995** *Baby Blue Jeans*	**1997** *Black Jeans*
1993 *Versus Uomo*	**1996** *Yellow Jeans*	**1997** *White Jeans*

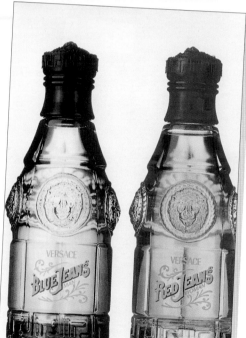

RED JEANS

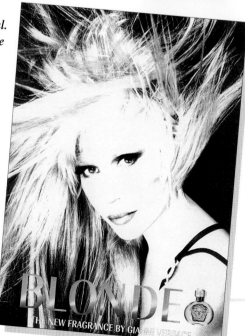

Launch: 1994

▲ Top notes: Redcurrant, Water-lily, Lilac stems, Freesia, Ylang-ylang

▲ Middle notes: Gardenia, Red peony, Jasmin, Violet

▲ Base notes: Sandalwood, Musk, Vanilla

Style: This light, carefree eau de toilette is designed for adventurous, liberated and self-confident young women. With an immediate red-fruit appeal followed by a heady floral bouquet on a lightly spicy base, it is the female half of the first duo in the *Jeans* collection.

Left: The 'soda-bottle' packaging of the Jeans *range expressed its youthful appeal. Right: Donatella Versace appeared as the 'face' of* Blonde.

BLONDE

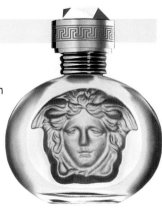

Launch: 1996

▲ Top notes: Violet leaves, Neroli

▲ Middle notes: Tuberose, Jasmin, Narcissus, Orange blossom

▲ Base notes: Orris, Broom, Everlasting flower

Style: This perfume was created in honour of Donatella Versace, who, in photographs by Richard Avedon, is its face . It is exuberant, sexy, strong and dynamic — like the archetypal Versace woman. The bottle, designed by Versace with Serge Mansau, has the famous Medusa logo in relief on the side.

JEAN PATOU

As a couturier, Jean Patou's designs were both elegant and casual, while the famous fragrances bearing his name are among the world's most luxurious.

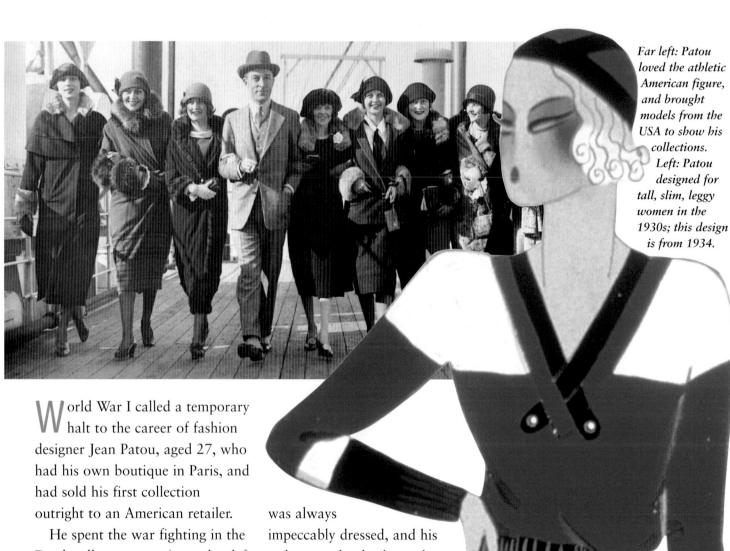

Far left: Patou loved the athletic American figure, and brought models from the USA to show his collections.
Left: Patou designed for tall, slim, leggy women in the 1930s; this design is from 1934.

World War I called a temporary halt to the career of fashion designer Jean Patou, aged 27, who had his own boutique in Paris, and had sold his first collection outright to an American retailer.

He spent the war fighting in the Dardanelles, an experience that left an indelible mark on him. Although he became a successful businessman in the 1920s, he determined to live life to the full.

THE ROARING TWENTIES

The tall, elegant Patou epitomized the spirit of the 1920s. He loved fast cars and beautiful women. Although he never married, he was said to have had many affairs. He was always impeccably dressed, and his style was relentlessly modern and chic. Between them, he and Chanel, with whom he enjoyed a lifelong friendly rivalry, invented the long, lean 1920s' silhouette. He favoured streamlined, simple shapes that could act as a blank canvas for jazzy geometric patterning. A perfectionist, he had cloth specially woven in his chosen colours. He was the first designer to be interested in accessories and pioneered the designer monogram. His adoring clients included the American movie stars Pola Negri, Louise Brooks and Mary Pickford, and a clutch of European princesses.

Patou targeted the modern young women who frequented resorts, such as Monte Carlo, Venice and Deauville, including rich American heiresses looking for aristocratic European husbands. They were active, liberated women who smoked, drove cars, swam, skied and played tennis and golf; they found Patou's casual but elegant sporty styles ideal. He designed knitwear, cruise clothes and bathing costumes, and dressed French tennis star Suzanne Lenglen on and off the court.

JOY TO THE WORLD

Like all French couturiers of the time, Patou courted the American market, and he launched *Joy*, still Patou's signature perfume, in 1930 to cosset his American clients after the Wall Street Crash. Called 'the costliest perfume in the world' by Elsa Maxwell, famous society

Above: At the 1921 Wimbledon tennis final, Suzanne Lenglen, one of Patou's favourite clients, won her third title in a white Patou pleated skirt that became a sportswear classic.

Right: Patou's love of long, slender lines was expressed as much in his evening wear as in the more casual styles that made his name. This gown is from 1931. Left: The house of Patou continues to create new fragrances 60 years after its founder's death; Un Amour de Patou was launched in 1998.

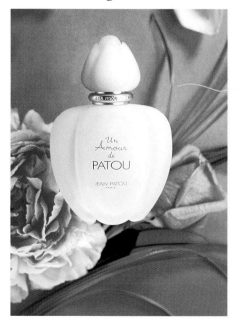

hostess and Patou's press agent, it was created by perfumer Henri Alméras, who was also responsible for six earlier Patou fragrances. It is a highly concentrated blend of rose de mai and Grasse jasmin, the most expensive ingredients.

MARKETING GENIUS

Patou had launched himself as a couturier perfumer in 1925 with three fragrances: the sensual, fruity *Amour Amour* for brunettes, the lighter floral *Que Sais-Je?* for blondes and spicy *Adieu Sagesse* for redheads. He had a genius for sales gimmicks; in 1929 he launched the first unisex perfume, *Le Sien* – the name can mean 'his' or 'hers'.

Le Normandie (1935) marked the maiden voyage of the luxury transatlantic liner. The striking ship-shaped bottle was designed by Louis Süe, a leading Art Deco

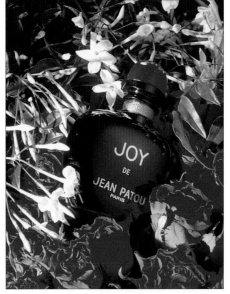

painter, and made by glass-makers Baccarat. *Vacances* celebrated the advent of paid holidays in 1936.

After Patou's untimely death that year, his brother-in-law, Raymond Barbas, headed the company and safeguarded its traditions of luxury, quality and taste. Commemorative fragrances continued to be issued, including *L'Heure Attendue* for the liberation of Paris in 1945.

Now run by Jean and Guy de Moüy, great-nephews of the

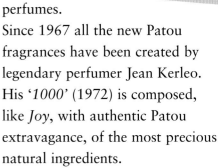

Right and left: From the beginning, Joy *made a virtue of its high cost and the distinctive Art Deco bottle in which it is still sold, although it is also available today in a red and black flaçon inspired by an oriental snuff bottle.*

founder, Patou still creates and makes its own perfumes.

Since 1967 all the new Patou fragrances have been created by legendary perfumer Jean Kerleo. His '*1000*' (1972) is composed, like *Joy*, with authentic Patou extravagance, of the most precious natural ingredients.

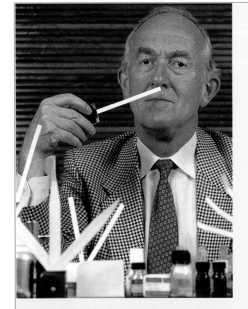

Jean Patou

PROFILE

1887 Jean Patou born in Normandy to a family of wealthy furriers.

1912 Opens his own boutique, Maison Parry, in Paris.

1914 Patou is called up into the French army when World War I breaks out.

1919 Presents first collection at 7 Rue Saint-Florentin, Paris.

1921 Suzanne Lenglen wins Wimbledon in a Patou tennis outfit.

1925 Creates his first three perfumes.

1930 Launches *Joy*, 'the costliest perfume in the world'.

1936 Jean Patou dies and is succeeded as chairman of the company by his brother-in-law, Raymond Barbas.

1967 Jean Kerleo (left) becomes perfumer at Patou.

1980 Jean de Moüy, Patou's great-nephew, takes over at Patou.

1984 Launches *Ma Collection*, a coffret of 12 classic fragrances in miniatures of the original flaçons.

PERFUME CHRONOLOGY

1925 *Amour Amour*	1929 *Le Sien*	1935 *Normandie*	1972 *'1000'*	1992 *Sublime*
1925 *Que Sais-Je?*	1930 *Joy*	1936 *Vacances*	1976 *Eau de Patou*	1995 *Voyageur*
1925 *Adieu Sagesse*	1930 *Cocktail*	1938 *Colony*	1980 *Patou pour*	1998 *Un Amour de*
1927 *Chaldée*	1932 *Invitation*	1946 *L'Heure Attendue*	*Homme*	*Patou*
1929 *Moment Suprême*	1933 *Divine Folie*	1964 *Caline*	1987 *Ma Liberté*	1999 *Patou Forever*

Jean Patou
C O L L E C T I O N

J O Y

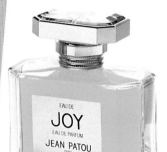

Launch: 1930
▲ Top notes: Damask rose, Tuberose, Ylang-ylang
▲ Middle notes: Jasmin, Rose de mai
▲ Base notes: Jasmin, Rose de mai
Style: The ultimate floral fragrance is a rich, concentrated blend of natural essences, principally jasmin from Grasse and rose de mai. An intense, almost intoxicating, and luxurious scent, it still comes in the original cut and polished crystal bottle designed by Louis S e, who also created the famous gold pine-cone -stoppered bottles used for earlier Patou perfumes. It was first formulated in 1930, but was not actually sold until 1932.

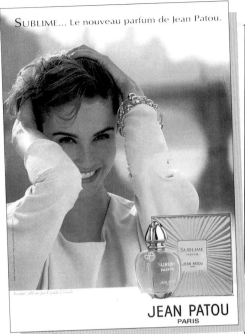

Above: The advertising for Sublime *speaks of summer in tones of gold and peach.*

'1 0 0 0'

Launch: 1972
▲ Top notes: Chinese osmanthus, Bulgarian rose
▲ Middle notes: Jasmin, Sweet violet, *Rosa centifolia*
▲ Base notes: Sandalwood, Patchouli
Style: Created by Jean Kerleo, this seductive, bold, floral-oriental perfume is even more expensive than *Joy*. The heady exoticism of osmanthus and jasmin, swathed in delicious roses and powdery violet, are underpinned by the warmth of precious tropical woods. It comes in a classic square-cut bottle with an engraved JP monogram and in an exquisite jade-coloured bottle inspired by a Chinese snuff box. The atomizer (right) fits neatly into a handbag.

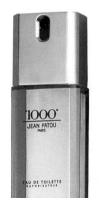

S U B L I M E

Launch: 1992
▲ Top notes: Orange blossom, Mandarin, Ylang-ylang
▲ Middle notes: Lily-of-the-valley, Rose, Jasmin, Orange blossom
▲ Base notes: Vetiver, Sandalwood, Oakmoss, Vanilla
Style: This sumptuous, fruity, Kerleo fragrance is warm and sensual, with a summery, floral heart and lightly spicy undertones. The curvaceous gold-topped bottle, suggestive of ripe fruit, was designed by Xavier Rousseau.

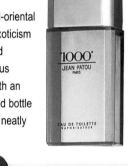

P A T O U   F O R E V E R

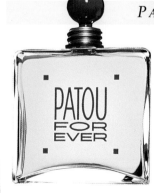

Launch: 1999
▲ Top notes: Raspberry, Pineapple, Melon, Balsam
▲ Middle notes: Rose, Lily-of-the-valley, Jasmin
▲ Base notes: Oakmoss, Vetiver, Sandalwood, Iris, Violet
Style: A silky, opulent fragrance bursting with the scents of warm, sun-ripened fruit and summer flowers, Kerleo s *Patou Forever* is sharpened by a lingering spiciness that is both sexy and sophisticated. The gorgeous bottle, with its plum-tinted glass stopper set in a gold band, is designed to enhance the scent s ambery colour. There is also a limited-edition fla on spray covered in burnished antique gold.

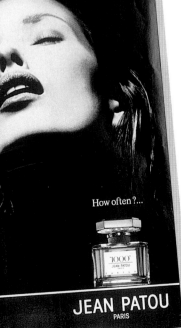

How often?...

Left and right: The advertising for '1000' is clearly sexual, while that for Patou Forever *makes an appeal to the discriminating woman.*

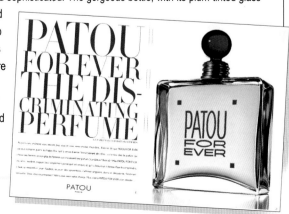

GUCCI

A new lease of life has been injected into this prestigious but strife-ridden fashion and perfume house by its current American director and designer Tom Ford.

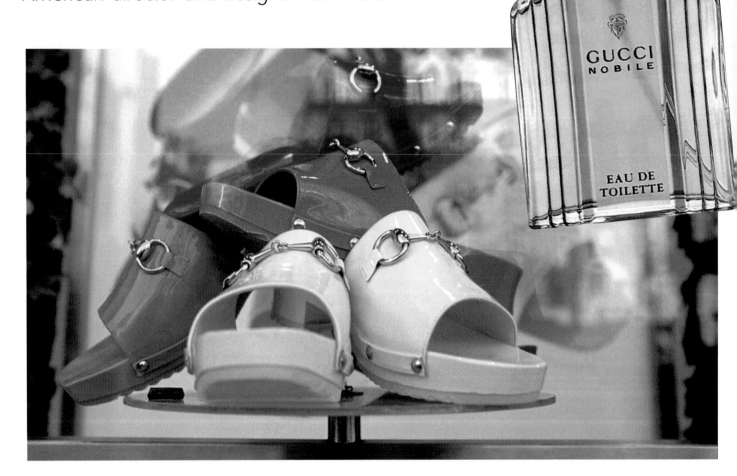

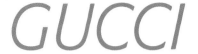

The 1995 shooting of Maurizio Gucci outside his Milan office by an assassin hired by his ex-wife, Patrizia, was the last and bloodiest act of vengeance in a Florentine family saga of intrigue, jealousy, violence, power, greed and betrayal. Fathers and sons, brothers and cousins had fought to control the multi-million dollar company founded by Maurizio's grandfather, Guccio Gucci, in 1906. Guccio first had the idea of a shop selling high-class leather goods when he was a waiter at London's Ritz Hotel. He realized that the guests' expensive leather luggage was a visible symbol of their wealth.

FIRST SHOP

Back in Florence, he opened a shop which made use of traditional Florentine leather-working skills to produce just such stylish items. In 1932 he designed the moccasin-inspired snaffle loafers that became

Above: Gucci made its name in the 1930s with classy casual shoes. These are modern updates.
Inset: Gucci Nobile, launched in 1988, was the company's second fragrance for men.

élite fashion icons for the next three decades, and in 1933 his son Aldo devised the intertwined GG monogram, the unmistakeable mark of quality on Gucci products.

Another Gucci classic, the canvas suitcase with green and red bands and leather trim, was Aldo's

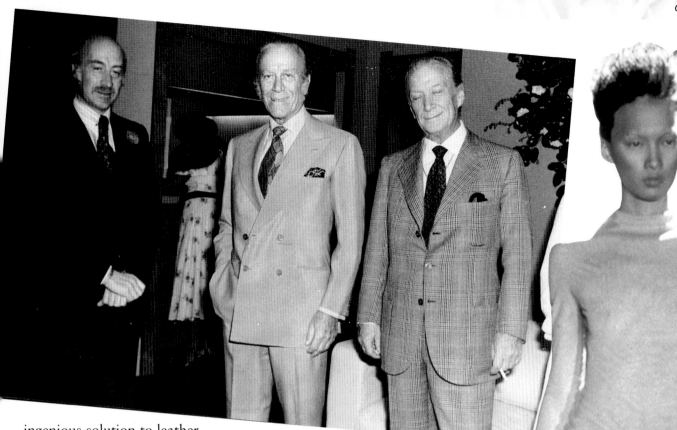

Above: Members of the ancient Florentine family included, from left, Paolo, Aldo and Rodolfo Gucci, photographed here in London.

ingenious solution to leather shortages in World War II.

In 1938, Aldo had opened a shop in Rome's ultra-fashionable Via Condotti which, after the war, became a mecca for rich American tourists looking for stylish trinkets.

NEW CHALLENGES

The company diversified into new products and the empire expanded, largely due to Aldo's drive and creative flair, but like his father – who died in 1953 – he expected obedience from his sons. Paolo, by this time chief designer, was especially rebellious. Aldo's brother Rodolfo and his son Maurizio also entered the picture.

A volatile brew of suspicion, resentment and frustration bubbled steadily through the 1970s, with fierce squabbles over, among other things, shares in the newly created Gucci Parfums. It finally boiled over in 1982 in a

notorious boardroom brawl, from which a bloodstained Paolo emerged, vowing vengeance.

Paolo waged protracted legal battles against the company, which ended in a jail sentence for his father. Rodolfo died and Maurizio, although accused of forging his father's will, inherited his share. Maurizio then ousted Aldo in a boardroom coup, but was himself removed by his new, more sedate, merchant-banking partners, Investcorps, in 1994.

During all this family strife, the company flourished. In 1985 it had over 150 shops world-wide and was reckoned to be worth around $800 million but, like all successful brands, it suffered from cheap imitations. Fighting these

Right: This sleek, stylish gown was featured in Gucci's 1997 autumn collection. The rebirth of the company as a leading fashion house followed the appointment of American Tom Ford as chief designer.

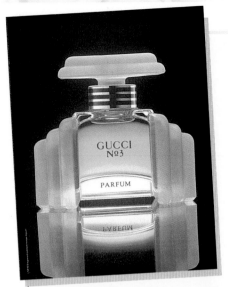

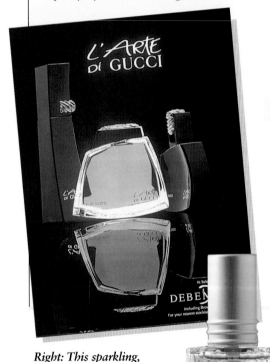

Above and below: These ads, simply of bottles mirrored on glass, reflect the traditional Gucci style of refinement and elegance.

Gucci

COLLECTION

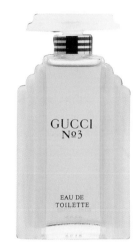

GUCCI NO 3

Launch: 1985
▲ Top notes: Lily-of-the-valley, Ylang-ylang, Coriander, Aldehydes
▲ Middle notes: Rose, Jasmin, Narcissus, Orris
▲ Base notes: Patchouli, Vetiver, Amber, Sandalwood, Musk, Balms
Style: Displaying all the refined chic of the traditional Gucci style, this classic floral-aldehyde perfume spells wealth and luxury, albeit discreetly, and with tantalizing hints of exoticism. The exquisitely elegant bottle designed by Peter Schmidt has slim columns of frosted glass set against clear, bright crystal.

L'ARTE DE GUCCI

Launch: 1992
▲ Top notes: Bergamot, Fruits, Camomile, Greens
▲ Middle notes: Rose, Jasmin, Lily-of-the-valley, Mimosa, Tuberose, Narcissus, Orris
▲ Base notes: Amber, Musk, Oakmoss, Patchouli, Leather, Vetiver
Style: This is a rich oriental perfume, with a sweet floral heart, which is packaged in a stylish, chocolate-coloured fla on.

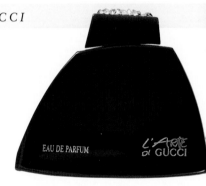

Right: This sparkling, youthful fragrance has been a popular success. It first appeared in 1982 but was relaunched in 1993.

and the endless family lawsuits became a financial drain. Valuable staff left the company and its prestigious aura began to falter.

In 1990, Maurizio appointed a new, American creative director,

who brought in the gifted young Texan Tom Ford as chief designer. He revitalized the label. The new style was sharp, hard-edged, modern and sexy.

Gucci Parfums was launched in 1974 with *Gucci No 1*, a classy, sophisticated floral scent that promoted the traditional Gucci values of quality and discreet elegance. Subsequent fragrances followed much the same style. The first signs of change came with *Accenti*, which

introduced original fruity notes. But it was *Envy*, the second fragrance since Tom Ford became creative director, that marked the decisive break. Upfront and unashamedly sensual, sharp and exciting, *Envy* is aimed at Gucci's new, young clientele. Both male and female fragrances are slightly androgynous, and the ice-cool green liquid in its starkly modern bottle provides a fitting symbolic contrast to Gucci's hot-blooded and sometimes inglorious past.

ACCENTI

Launch: 1995

▲ Top notes: Davana (Indian artemisia), Blackcurrant, Mandarin

▲ Middle notes: Rose, Jasmin, Clove, Lily-of-the-valley

▲ Base notes: Vetiver, Sandalwood, Patchouli, Vanilla, Tonka bean, Peach, Raspberry

Style: This is an elegant, floral-fruity fragrance full of fresh, subtle contrasts, expressing romance and femininity in a thoroughly modern way. It was created by perfumers Florasynth and is packaged in a classy, square-cut bottle designed by Alain de Mourgues.

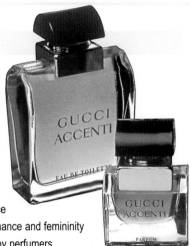

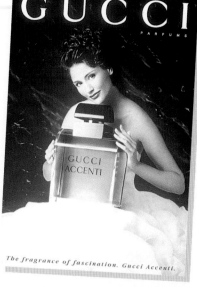

The fragrance of fascination. Gucci Accenti.

ENVY

Launch: 1997

▲ Top notes: Hyacinth, Magnolia, Green notes

▲ Middle notes: Lily-of-the-valley, Jasmin, Violet

▲ Base notes: Iris, Precious woods, Musk

Style: Created by perfumer Maurice Roucel, this breakthrough fragrance expresses the new, modern Gucci identity. It is an overtly seductive fragrance composed of intensely sensual flower scents with lightly piercing green notes, inspired by the elusive scent of the vine flower. The stunning minimalist bottle is reminiscent of a modernist skyscraper, a reflection perhaps of Tom Ford s architectural training.

Above and below: Under Tom Ford's direction, Gucci's image has become more upfront and overtly sexual, notably in the highly charged advertisement for Envy.

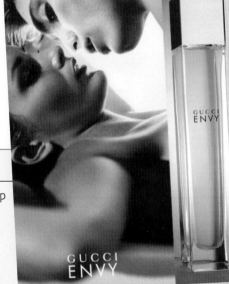

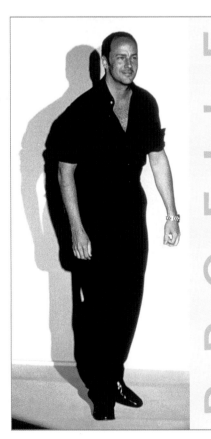

PROFILE

Gucci

1906	Guccio Gucci founds saddlery and leather shop in Florence.
1932	Famous snaffle loafers designed by Guccio.
1938	Guccio's son Aldo opens shop in Rome.
1953	First US Gucci shop opens in Fifth Avenue, New York.
1953	Aldo takes over as head of Gucci.
1974	Launch of first perfume, *Gucci No 1*.
1982	Family squabbles culminate in boardroom brawl; Aldo's son Paolo ousted.
1983	Rodolfo dies; son Maurizio accused of forging his will.
1984	Maurizio deposes Aldo in boardroom coup.
1986	Aldo imprisoned in the US for tax evasion.
1989	Maurizio becomes Gucci president.
1990	Tom Ford (left) joins Gucci as chief designer.
1993	Investicorp takes over Gucci; Maurizio removed.
1994	Tom Ford becomes creative director.
1995	Maurizio murdered; Tom Ford's acclaimed collection marks renaissance of Gucci.
1998	Maurizio's wife Patrizia sentenced to 29 years for ordering the murder of her husband.

PERFUME CHRONOLOGY

1974	*Gucci No 1*
1976	*Gucci pour Homme*
1982	*Eau de Gucci*
1985	*Gucci No 3*
1988	*Gucci Nobile*
1992	*L'Arte de Gucci*
1995	*Accenti*
1997	*Envy*
1998	*Envy For Men*

ISSEY MIYAKE

Japan's top designer, Issey Miyake, brings an exotic elegance and a cool intelligence to Parisian couture and applies the same qualities to his innovative perfumes.

Above: Miyake's flair for shape and colour is also expressed in the packaging of his fragrances; this summer version of L'Eau d'Issey keeps the bottle shape but introduces green, yellow and blue to symbolize the extra ingredients of kiwi, citrus and mint.

Above: At their best, Miyake's designs are a stunning combination of the futuristic and the traditional; the full lines of the garments come to life on the wearer, and move with her.

Issey Miyake was born in Hiroshima in 1938. He was just six years old, and bicycling to school, when the first atomic bomb was dropped on the city. More than 300,000 people died in the first few days, and young Issey lost almost all of his family.

Although he rarely talks of this experience and his manner is warm and jovial, there is, unsurprisingly, something essentially serious about Issey Miyake. His clothes might be exuberant and are rarely sombre, but they are never frivolous. He is the thinking woman's couturier, the universally acknowledged emperor of intellectual chic.

After training as a graphic designer in Tokyo, in 1965 he made a pilgrimage to Paris, where he honed his technique with Guy Laroche and Givenchy. The strait-laced French attitudes to couture were not to his taste; he preferred London, where the 1960s fashion revolution was in full swing.

RETURN TO TOKYO

After a brief stint in New York with Geoffrey Beene, the progressive designer of elegant sportswear, he returned to his cultural and aesthetic roots in Tokyo, where he founded the Miyake Design Studio (MDS). He shows twice yearly in Paris, mounts exhibitions in Europe and the USA and has built up a global chain of more than 150 shops. However, his working base and spiritual home remain in Japan, where he is a national hero, employing a devoted group of young designers and technicians, who help him realize his extraordinary vision.

PARADOXICAL CLOTHING

Miyake's work is full of paradoxes: it is both innovative and traditional, minimalist and complex, and accessible and avant-garde. Moulded plastic torsos and coiled wire bustiers look like pieces of modern sculpture; woven rattan bodices recall samurai body armour, while equally his swathed, cloak-like garments could be the mantles of Buddhist priests or costumes for *Star Wars*.

He finds Japanese costumes and textiles an inexhaustible source of inspiration for fabrics, shapes and structures. His first major collection made use of *sashiko*, the quilted cottons worn by fishermen; indigo dyes, *kasuri* (ikat) and *shibori* (tie-dyed) fabrics appear frequently.

Because Miyake's shapes are simple, the fabric is crucial. His clothes are rarely shaped to the body, tending to be loose, layered and voluminous; they are wrapped, folded, tucked and tied rather than fastened with buttons and zips. The fabric itself may be ruched, crushed, crinkled, crumpled or pleated.

To Miyake, 'fabric' does not have to mean cloth; he uses metal, wire mesh, tinfoil, rubber, straw, bamboo and synthetics of all kinds.

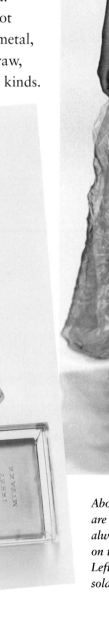

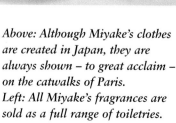

Above: Although Miyake's clothes are created in Japan, they are always shown – to great acclaim – on the catwalks of Paris.
Left: All Miyake's fragrances are sold as a full range of toiletries.

Issey Miyake

1938 Issey Miyake born in Hiroshima, Japan.
1963 Shows first collection in Tokyo.
1965 Works in Paris for Givenchy and Guy Laroche
1968 Goes to New York to work for Geoffrey Beene.
1970 Founds Miyake Design Studio (MDS) in Tokyo.
1973 Begins presenting twice-yearly collections in Paris.
1976 Presents collections in Osaka and Tokyo.
1977 Presents collections in Tokyo and Kyoto.
1983 Exhibition 'Issey Miyake Spectacle Bodyworks' in Japan and USA.
1984 Wins Council of Fashion Designers of America award.
1985 Exhibition 'Issey Miyake Fashion without Taboos' at the V&A, London.
1989 Wins Mainichi Fashion Grand Prix; puts on first 'Pleats' show.
1992 Miyake (below) launches first perfume, *L'Eau d'Issey*.
1996 Starts the Guest Artist series with Yasumasa Marimura.
1997 Show with Inokuma and Isami Noguchi at Museum of Contemporary Art in Shikoku.
1998-9 Exhibition 'Issey Miyake Making Things' at the Fondation Cartier pour l'Art Contemporain in Paris.

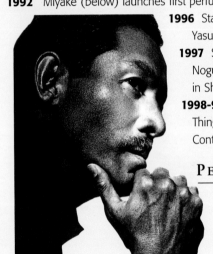

PERFUME CHRONOLOGY

1992 *L'Eau d'Issey*
1994 *L'Eau d'Issey pour Homme*
1998 *Le Feu d'Issey*

He once made a bat-winged, hooded coat from the oiled ochre paper usually seen on Japanese parasols.

He also constantly redefines the concept of clothing. In 1999, for example, he launched APOC, 'a piece of cloth' designed to be cut by the wearer to make a variety of garments – skirt, dress, hat, trousers or bikini – with choice of hemline, sleeve length and so on. This way, rather than impose his idea on the wearer, he includes her in the creative process.

FIRST FRAGRANCE

When the time came to launch a fragrance, he adopted a similar approach. In fact, his first feeling was that he positively disliked perfume. Rather than a powerful

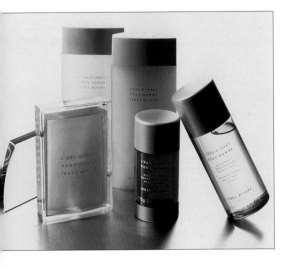

Left: L'Eau d'Issey pour Homme *is a livelier, more herby and distinctly less floral version of the original feminine fragrance.*

Issey Miyake
COLLECTION

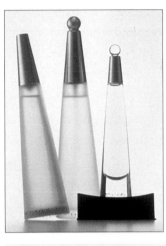

L'EAU D'ISSEY

Launch: 1992

▲ Top notes: Lotus, Freesia, Cyclamen, Rosewat[...]
▲ Middle notes: Peony, Carnation, Water-lily
▲ Base notes: Musk, Ambrette, Tuberose, Osmanthus, Precious woods

Style: This simple, yet sophisticated fragrance blen[...] delicate, flowery scents with the sparkling freshnes[...] splashing water and the earthy smells of rain-soake[...] springtime woods. A supremely elegant, frosty bottl[...] with a water droplet cap, designed by Alain Mourgu[...] and Fabien Baron, continues the theme. Limited edition summer fragrances are launched every yea[...] The 1999 version includes the aromachological essences of citrus, kiwi and mint to revitalize the bo[...] boost optimism and soothe the spirit.

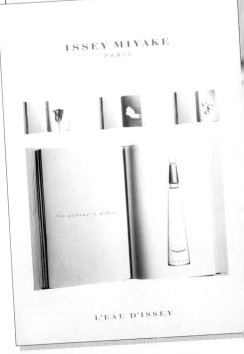

L'EAU D'ISSEY POUR HOMME

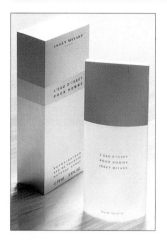

Launch: 1994

▲ Top notes: Lemon verbena, Coriander, Sage, Yuzu fruit, Mandarin

▲ Middle notes: Water-lily, Cinnamon, Nutmeg, Saffron, Geranium, Mint, Sandalwood, Cedar

▲ Base notes: Amber, Musk

Style: This is a more bubbly, agile and energetic interpretation of the scent of water than its counterpart for women, with invigorating, bracing top notes, a more exotic spicy heart, and the sensuous, musky smell of rich, moist, dark earth at the base. The packaging includes a variety of irresistible minimalist objects, including an ingenious Zippo-style, brushed-steel travel spray and a shockproof, rubberized toilet bag — shaped like a space capsule — which holds fragrance and matching shampoo, after-shave, body gel and other accessories.

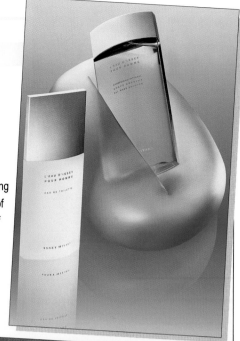

LE FEU D'ISSEY

Launch: 1998

▲ Top notes: Bulgarian rose, Coriander leaves

▲ Middle notes: Sichuan pepper, Golden Japanese lily

▲ Base notes: Guaiac wood, Milky amber, Benzoin, Amber

Style: Vibrant, warm, optimistic and emotional, this floral-spicy-woody *eau de toilette* by Jacques Cavallier is a complete contrast to the coolness of his other creation, *L Eau d Issey*. It combines vitality and seductiveness and calmness and strength, but the overall feeling is ultra-feminine and completely, unashamedly pleasurable. The tactile spherical container, designed by Gw na l Nicolas, is made of PCTA Waterclear, a special synthetic material that looks like glass but is warm to the touch. It is made up of two burnt orange cones inside a transparent sphere, and includes a cleverly-constructed push-button catch. The range also includes a bath gel and body lotion that incorporate ginseng, tea-tree oil and juniper, and are packaged in phosphorescent green and orange bottles .

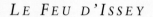

Right, above right and opposite lower right: The ads for all three Miyake fragrances share the same basic style, with a single base colour, a photo of the pack and very few words. This minimalist approach, with its bold, simple shapes and elegant restraint, is entirely in accord with Miyake's philosophy of design.

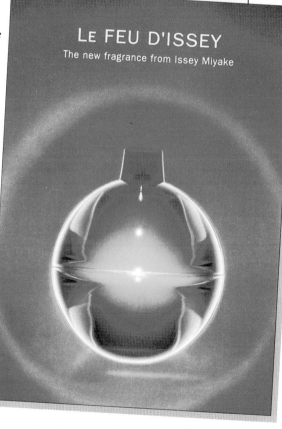

scent, he wanted something 'that didn't smell at all' but, like his clothes, would move to suit the woman wearing it, embracing rather than overwhelming her – a perfume with 'the fragrance of dew and rain falling on plants' and the purity, cleanness and freshness of water.

This challenge was accepted by master-perfumer Jacques Cavallier of Firmenich. In 1992 he came up

with *L'Eau d'Issey*, a scent that was delicate, very feminine and full of vitality, but deep and lasting. New synthetic ozonic notes evoked sparkling streams and waterfalls rather than the salty tang of the sea.

A male version followed in 1994, and then came the second of his elemental fragrances, *Le Feu d'Issey*, a floral-spicy-woody blend

that is warm, dynamic and radiates energy. 'The fire of life' had literally succeeded 'the water of life' ('issey' in Japanese means 'life'). This makes it an appropriate name for a someone who has been part of the renewal of Japanese culture since the terrible destruction of August 1945.

NINA RICCI

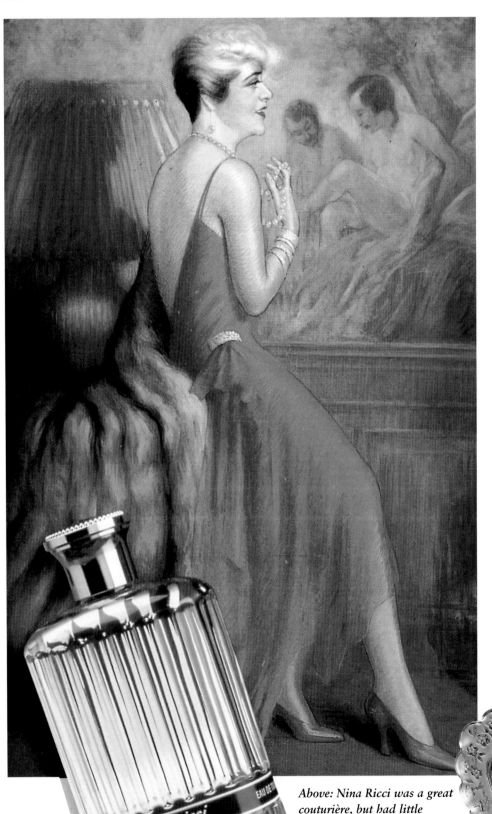

Above: Nina Ricci was a great couturière, but had little interest in perfume. Fragrances such as Signoricci (left) and Coeur-Joie (right) were the passion of her son Robert.

With the encouragement and active partnership of her son, Italian-born Nina Ricci set up a Parisian fashion and fragrance house renowned for its style and elegance.

In 1932 Nina Ricci was 49, and had virtually retired to a life of luxury and unaccustomed leisure with her second husband, wealthy industrialist Gaston Morel. Her career as a successful designer of elegant clothes for wealthy women seemed over, but its most glittering period was yet to begin.

ITALIAN ORIGINS

Nina Ricci was born Maria Nielli in Turin in 1883. In 1895 she went to France with her elder sister to seek her fortune, and at 13 was apprenticed to a dressmaker. A mix of talent, ambition and hard work meant that four years later she was running the workshop, and at 22 she was chief designer. She met and married Luigi Ricci, and in 1905 their son Robert was born. The marriage was not a success. Luigi

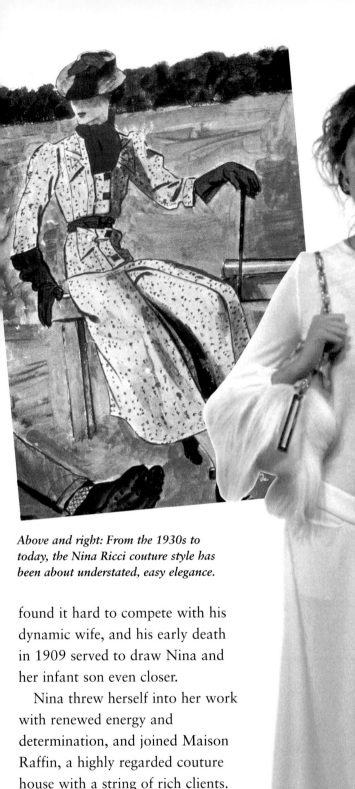

Above and right: From the 1930s to today, the Nina Ricci couture style has been about understated, easy elegance.

found it hard to compete with his dynamic wife, and his early death in 1909 served to draw Nina and her infant son even closer.

Nina threw herself into her work with renewed energy and determination, and joined Maison Raffin, a highly regarded couture house with a string of rich clients. She was there for more than 20 years, having carved out her own domain within the firm, with her own workshops, staff and clients.

She was known for producing flattering, fashionable clothes that were elegant and even glamorous, but not too daring. They were beautifully cut, impeccably made and usually about a third of the price of a Schiaparelli or Lanvin –

virtues well appreciated by a traditional bourgeois clientele looking for quality and good value.

In 1929 Maison Raffin closed, and Nina devoted herself to the good life, kept busy with her three homes, her jewellery – she had a huge collection of pearls – and her fast cars, especially her famous white Cadillac.

OUT OF RETIREMENT

Nina had no need to work, and did not expect to do so, but her son changed her mind. Robert Ricci had inherited her drive and ambition; he was running his own advertising agency when they joined forces to found their own couture and perfume house, Maison Nina Ricci. He controlled the visual side of the new company, involving artists, such as Christian Bérard and Marc Lalique, in the design of ads, packaging and bottles.

Robert created the company as a kind of homage to his mother, and it was very much in her image. A totally feminine house-style reflected charm, refinement and unthreatening elegance in a quietly seductive way. It was the epitome of timeless Parisian chic – grown-up clothes for grown-up women.

Nina was a brilliant cutter; she would virtually sculpt the cloth to create a romantic ideal of femininity – more dream than reality – but immensely appealing.

The designers who succeeded Nina remained true to that spirit, and when Robert decided to produce perfumes, he favoured a gentle, rather romantic style. Perfume became a passion for him. 'It is music for the emotions,' he claimed. 'It speaks to the soul.' His first fragrance, *Coeur-Joie* (1946), celebrated the joy of victory after World War II.

The bottle, designed by Marc Lalique, was an open crystal heart engraved with flowers. Lalique

Right: The close association between the Ricci and Lalique families produced several remarkably beautiful flaçons.

designed exclusively for Ricci and his friend Robert; his most famous creation was for Ricci's all-time classic *L'Air du Temps* (1948), with a swirl of clear crystal stoppered by a pair of frosty entwined doves – symbols of both love and peace.

EXPANDING RANGE

Other scents followed, some of which are still available: among them the chypre-style *Fille d'Eve* and *Fleur de Fleurs*, a light, floral, daytime scent.

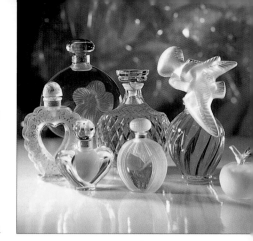

In 1987 came Robert Ricci's other masterpiece, *Nina*, named in testament to the bond of mutual love, respect and admiration that had powered the progress of one of the world's top fashion, perfume and cosmetics companies. Nina Ricci continues to flourish, with thoroughly modern scents such as *Deci Delà* and *Les Belles de Ricci*.

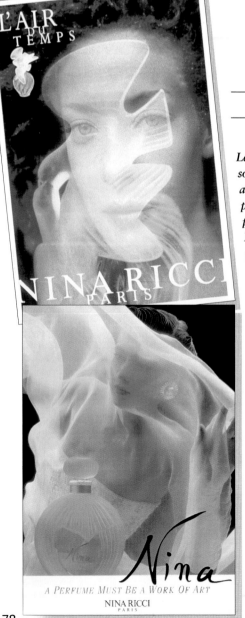

L'AIR DU TEMPS

NINA RICCI
PARIS

Nina

A PERFUME MUST BE A WORK OF ART
NINA RICCI
PARIS

Nina Ricci
COLLECTION

Left and below: The sometimes gauzy advertising photographs used to promote classic Nina Ricci fragrances express a kind of soft-focus femininity in keeping with the company's traditional image.

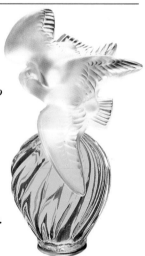

L'AIR DU TEMPS

Launch: 1948
▲ Top notes: Bergamot, Carnation, Rose
▲ Middle notes: Gardenia, Jasmin, Rose, Ylang-ylang
▲ Base notes: Musk, Orris, Sandalwood
Style: This gloriously lively, happy-ever-after floral perfum was designed, much like Dior s New Look, to reflect the jo and optimism of the post-war period — the spirit of the tim in its name. This tender, sweet, romantic fragrance has si become a dazzlingly successful classic. Never overpowering, it blends with the individual scent of the ski to make something unique for each woman wearing it. Its most famous bottle, designed by Marc Lalique and launch in 1958, carries a stopper of two entwined doves billing ar cooing. The 1951 box was shaped like a domed birdcage and covered in pleated yellow silk; it could be lit up by a battery in an accompanying purse.

NINA

Launch: 1987
▲ Top notes: Bergamot, Cassia buds, Basil
▲ Middle notes: Jasmin, Mimosa, Rose, Iris, Violet, Ylang-ylang, Orange blossom
▲ Base notes: Sandalwood, Vetiver, Marigold, Blackcurrant
Style: Created by Robert Ricci with perfumer Christian Vacchiano as a homage to his mother, this deeply pleasurable fragrance uses mostly natural ingredients to harmonize the warm sensuality of roses and jasmin with exotic floral scents and woody, fruity notes. The frosted glass bottle, which echoes the sculpted drapery of Nina s clothes, was designed by Marie-Claude Lalique, daughter of Marc and grand-daughter of the famous glassmaker and jeweller Ren Lalique.

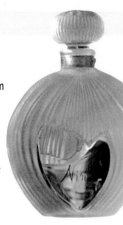

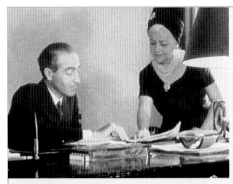

Nina Ricci

1883 Maria Nielli born in Turin, Italy.
1896 Apprenticed to a dressmaker in Monte Carlo.
1897 Moves to Paris.
1904 Marries jeweller Luigi Ricci.
1905 Robert Ricci is born.
1908 Nina joins Maison Raffin as a designer; stays there for 20 years.
1932 Sets up own couture house in the Boulevard des Capucines, Paris, with Robert.
1945 Robert (left, with his mother) becomes official director.
1946 Launches first fragrance, *Coeur-Joie*.
1970 Nina Ricci dies.
1979 The company moves its headquarters to Avenue Montaigne, Paris's most prestigious couture quarter.
1987 Launch of *Nina*, with a gala evening at the Opèra Garnier.
1989 Robert Ricci dies.
1992 House of Ricci creates its first cosmetic line, Le Teint Ricci.
1998 Fiftieth birthday celebrations for *L'Air du Temps*.
1998 Becomes part of the PUIG group of companies.

PERFUME CHRONOLOGY

1946	*Coeur-Joie*	**1974**	*Farouche*
1948	*L'Air du Temps*	**1975**	*Signoricci 2*
1949	*Douce*	**1980**	*Eau de Fleurs*
1952	*Fille d'Eve*	**1984**	*Phileas*
1961	*Capricci*	**1987**	*Nina*
1965	*Signoricci 1*	**1989**	*Ricci Club*
1967	*Mademoiselle Ricci*	**1994**	*Deci Delà*
1971	*Bigarade*	**1996**	*Les Belles de Ricci*

DECI DELÀ

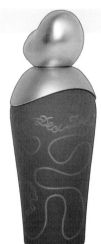

Launch: 1994
▲ Top notes: Peach, Raspberry, Redcurrant, Boronia, Osmanthus
▲ Middle notes: Rose de mai, Sweet pea, Freesia, Hazelnut
▲ Base notes: Sandalwood, Patchouli, Oakmoss, Cambodian agarwood, Balsam, Cypress, Cedar

Style: The intoxicating scent of sweet red raspberries, sun-warmed peaches and ripe apricots (from the osmanthus) are followed by the intensity of freesia and rose de mai and subtle, sweet pea notes. These are underpinned with voluptuous precious woods and oakmoss in this thoroughly modern, luscious, fruity-floral fragrance with over 100 mainly natural ingredients. The curvaceous, arty bottle in opalescent glass comes in three fruity colours — cherry, mandarin and raspberry — and is topped by a matt gold, cloud-shaped collar and stopper.

LES BELLES DE RICCI

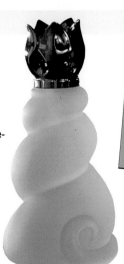

Launch: 1996
▲ Top notes: Mint, Basil, Tomato (leaf, flower and fruit)
▲ Middle notes: Wisteria, Magnolia, Nasturtium, Freesia
▲ Base notes: Raspberry, Figwood, Myrrh, Cedar, Cypress

Style: The original *Les Belles de Ricci* is basically a light and youthful fragrance with an immediate, spontaneous appeal, sparkling with good-to-be-alive freshness and full of easy-going fun. In April 1999, the name *Les Belles de Ricci* was expanded into an umbrella term for three bright and breezy *eaux de toilette* formulated to match the changing moods of young women. The original version in the green bottle, renamed Liberty Fizz, was joined by the romantic Almond Amour in a matching blue bottle, with strong almond and vanilla notes and floral touches, and the sensual fragrance, Spicy Delight, with citrus and spices in an orange bottle.

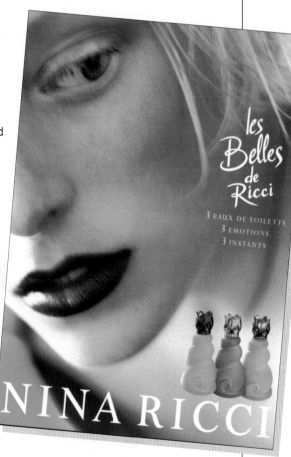

Above: Les Belles de Ricci *is aimed at a more youthful market than other Nina Ricci fragrances, and this is reflected in a bolder, more assertive advertising style.*

RALPH LAUREN

Ralph Lauren's creations celebrate the American dream of plenty; his fragrances, like his clothes, are about elegance and ivy-league lifestyles.

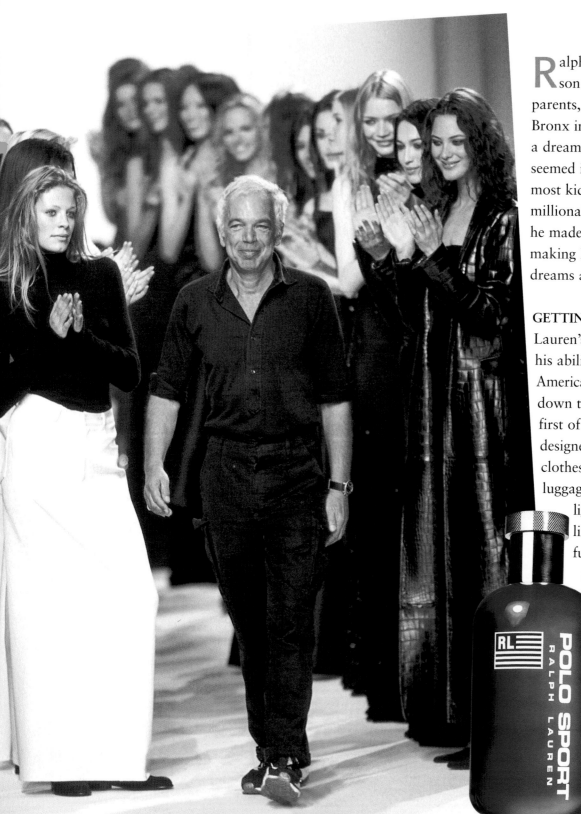

Ralph Lifschitz, the youngest son of Russian immigrant parents, was born in New York's Bronx in 1939. Young Ralph was a dreamer of what must have seemed impossible dreams. Like most kids, he wanted to be a millionaire, but unlike most kids, he made it, and he made it by making his own and other people's dreams a reality.

GETTING A LIFE

Lauren's huge success is based on his ability to package a bundle of American aspirational fantasies down to the utmost detail. The first of the 'fashion as lifestyle' designers, he provides not only clothes, underwear, shoes, luggage and fragrance, but also lighting, bed and table linen, glassware, crockery, furniture and even paint for the walls.

In a career of nearly 40 years, he has returned time and

Left: Lauren's evocation of aspirational lifestyles in his clothes and fragrances extends from the casual elegance of the 1920s to the work-out culture of today. Both sport and wealth are symbolized in his Polo trademark.

again to the seductive vision of an earlier golden age, spruced up and romanticized for the modern world. The American myths of ranchers and cowboys were expressed in his 1970s' 'prairie look', and he has also evoked the equivalent English myth of the oak-panelled country house with ancestor portraits.

PICKING POLO

Early in his career Lauren worked for Brooks Brothers, pioneers of US preppie clothes. Their famous button-down-collar shirt was based on those worn by European players of polo, the upper-class sport of kings and princes.

When he set up his own company in 1967, he called it Polo because it seemed 'moneyed and stylish'. His first line of wide 'kipper' ties was such a success that he borrowed $50,000 to design a collection of 'Gatsby' clothes to go with the ties, inspired by the man-about-town styles of the 1920s and '30s. Four years later, he could have repaid the loan 15 times over.

WOMENSWEAR

His switch to womenswear followed the same principles of timeless elegance. An early triumph was the 'Annie Hall' look (he designed Diane Keaton's clothes for the film), in which he scaled down his men's tailored jackets, trousers, shirts, waistcoats and trilby hats for an easy-to-wear, casual stylishness that is still hugely popular.

Creating a long-lasting, classic style was always more important

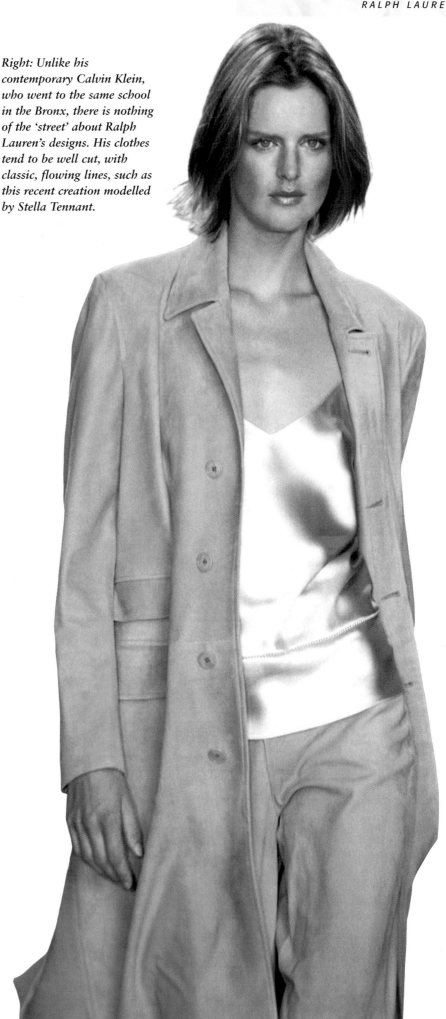

Right: Unlike his contemporary Calvin Klein, who went to the same school in the Bronx, there is nothing of the 'street' about Ralph Lauren's designs. His clothes tend to be well cut, with classic, flowing lines, such as this recent creation modelled by Stella Tennant.

to Lauren than the instant fix of fashion. He took the same view of his fragrances. Each was designed to enhance and fulfil aspects of his enduring visions.

FRAGRANCE STYLES

His first perfumes reflect his attraction to the country-house tradition: *Lauren* is totally feminine in a coolly elegant way, with a clean, fresh fruitiness in the top notes and a soft floral heart, while *Polo* is distinctively masculine, a chypre-style fragrance redolent of rough tweeds and old leather, and presented in hip-flask bottles.

Chaps (1979), *Tuxedo* (1979) and *Safari* (1990) conjure similarly vivid images. With *Polo Sport* (1994) and *Polo Sport Woman* (1996) he expresses his other loves – for sport, sporting images and sportswear. Both are clean,

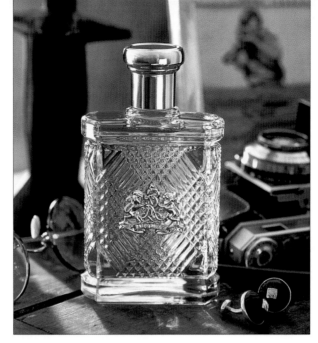

Left: The faceted flaçon for Safari for Men *is in the shape of a hip flask. The applied metal crest adds to the image of a wealthy international traveller of the 1930s and 1940s; all Lauren's 'lifestyle creations' tend to be tied to a particular time, as well as to a place and way of life.*

exhilarating scents that tune into the 1990s' enthusiasm for physical fitness and athleticism.

His 1999 perfume, *Romance*, in a way evokes his entire career and his approach to life. He is a clever businessman and a brilliantly intuitive designer, who has made a fortune selling romantic visions of the good life. These are not merely cynical marketing ploys, but his own aspirations – the dreams of a

Bronx boy who started work at 15 and shared a bedroom with his brother until he was 23.

Even now, happily married to the same woman for 35 years, with three successful children, five fabulous homes and a fashion empire with annual revenues of over $1 billion, he is still a driven man, still searching for 'the ultimate dream'. And if Ralph Lauren can imagine it, he will make it come true.

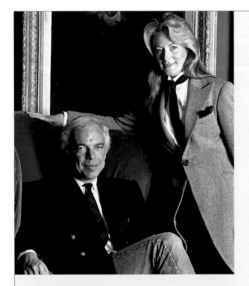

PERFUME CHRONOLOGY

1978 *Lauren*	**1992** *Safari for Men*
1978 *Polo for Men*	**1994** *Polo Sport*
1979 *Chaps*	**1996** *Polo Sport Woman*
1979 *Tuxedo*	**1998** *Extreme Polo Sport*
1990 *Safari*	**1999** *Romance*

PROFILE

Ralph Lauren

1939	Ralph Lifschitz born on 14 October in the Bronx, New York.
1968	Establishes menswear company, Polo by Ralph Lauren.
1970	Wins first of seven Coty American Fashion Critics Awards.
1971	Opens the first Polo store in Beverly Hills; founds Ralph Lauren Womenswear.
1972	Launches line of lower-priced menswear, Chaps.
1974	Designs costumes for Robert Redford in *The Great Gatsby*.
1977	Designs costumes for *Annie Hall*.
1978	Lauren (left, with his wife) launches Polo for Boys and first fragrance, *Lauren*.
1981	Opens first international store in London; wins Coty Hall of Fame award.
1983	Launches the Ralph Lauren Home Collection.
1986	Opens flagship store in the Rhinelander mansion on Madison Avenue.
1992	Wins Lifetime Achievement Award from the Council of Fashion Designers of America.
1995	Establishes the Ralph Lauren Womenswear Company.
1996	Launches Polo Jeans, Polo Sport Woman Collection and line of lower-priced womenswear, Lauren.
1997	Receives Council of Fashion Designers of America award for Menswear Designer of the Year.
1999	Opens new flagship store at 1 New Bond Street, London.

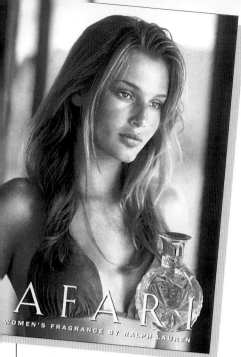

Ralph Lauren
C O L L E C T I O N

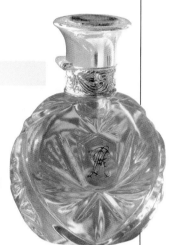

S A F A R I

Launch: 1990

▲ Top notes: Marigold, Jonquil, Mandarin

▲ Middle notes: Narcissus, Broom, Rose, Jasmin, Iris, Orange blossom

▲ Base notes: Sandalwood, Amber, Patchouli, Vetiver, Cedar

Style: This award-winning, green-floral fragrance with an intensely sensual heart has distinctly warm, lightly exotic undertones and is both sophisticated and womanly. The cut-glass bottle with silver monogrammed top and the mock crocodile box lined with ivory damask hark back to an earlier, classier age of stylish comfort and casual elegance.

P O L O   S P O R T   W O M A N

Launch: 1996

▲ Top Notes: Water mint, Pennyroyal, Citrus, Orange flower, Eucalyptus, Melon

▲ Middle notes: Poppy, Freesia, Lily, Ylang-ylang, Ginger, Nutmeg

▲ Base notes: Sandalwood, Cedar, Musk

Style: A fragrance designed to evoke femininity, grace and strength, and enhance the architecture of a beautiful body, *Polo Sport Woman* is designed for self-assured, body-conscious women keen on sports and physical fitness. It is a translucent floral scent that is both energizing and cooling, enveloped in soothing, warm and woody undertones. There is a range of complementary skincare products infused with sea organics , a blend of marine ingredients, including kelp and algae, which help invigorate, tone and pamper the skin.

E X T R E M E   P O L O   S P O R T

Launch: 1998

▲ Top notes: Black pepper oil, Bergamot, Rosewood, Juniper, Nutmeg, Coriander, Mint

▲ Middle notes: Clary sage, Champaca wood, Cypress, Cardamom

▲ Base notes: Sandalwood, Musk, Elemi

Style: A unisex eau de toilette that is more masculine than feminine, *Extreme Polo Sport* is designed for the more adventurous athletes, accustomed to pushing themselves and their bodies to the limits. It is an exhilarating, almost aggressive, woody-spicy fragrance with a rush of powerful peppery, lemon notes, both uplifting and energizing, which are softened by the warmth of nutmeg and refreshed by mint. Juniper and champaca wood reduce anxiety, while cardamom, clary sage, sandalwood and elemi are tonics and stimulants.

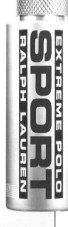

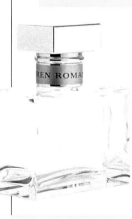

Right, top left and centre left: All the campaigns for Lauren perfumes feature versions of the Lauren woman – blonde and full lipped with high cheekbones.

R O M A N C E

Launch: 1999

▲ Top notes: Ginger, Lychee, Marigold, Freesia, Camomile oil, Sungoddess rose

▲ Middle notes: Day lily, White violet, Paradisone, Lotus flower

▲ Base notes: Patchouli, Oakmoss, Skin musk 2000, Exotic woods

Style: This sensuously feminine, woody-floral perfume, packed in an understated, smooth, crystal-clear bottle and silver-accented box with soft pink panels, attempts to evoke the timeless essence of romance. Its playful, effervescent blend of sweet-scented garden flowers and exotics is given depth and richness by patchouli, oakmoss and musk and manages to be both tender and elegant, simple and refined.

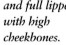

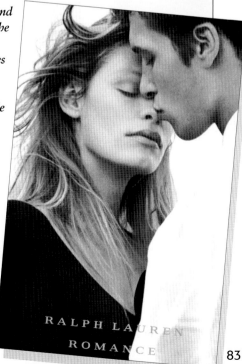

83

REVLON

The firm founded by the Revson brothers began by selling make-up, but soon took up the cudgels to challenge the great names of the American beauty business, a rivalry that spilled over into the fragrance market.

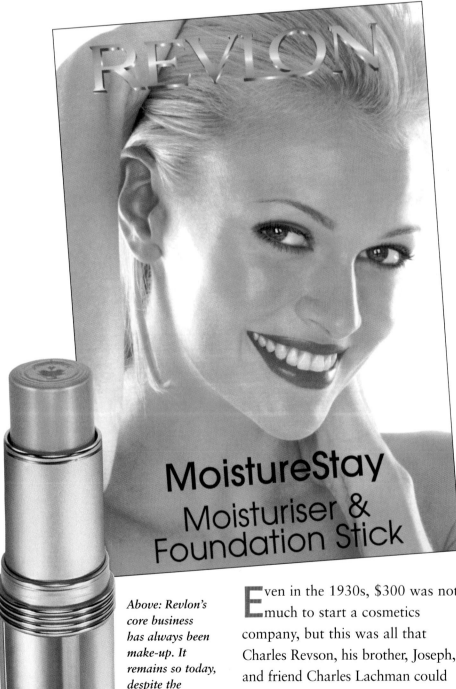

MoistureStay
Moisturiser &
Foundation Stick

Above: Revlon's core business has always been make-up. It remains so today, despite the success of its fragrance lines – especially Charlie.

Even in the 1930s, $300 was not much to start a cosmetics company, but this was all that Charles Revson, his brother, Joseph, and friend Charles Lachman could raise. It was enough. Within 10 years they had built a company to rival those of Estée Lauder, Helena Rubinstein and Elizabeth Arden. These three doyennes of the beauty business were furious. Arden always referred acidly to Revson as 'that man' – he retaliated by giving the tag to a perfume – while to Rubinstein he was 'the nail man', a dismissive reference to the nail varnish that made the company's name.

FILLING A GAP

Charles Revson had a real flair for marketing, for spotting gaps or selling an established product in a fresh way. Revlon's new nail lacquer was revolutionary, and he made the most of it. Previously, women had worn clear varnish in natural pink or beige, but chemist Lachman found a way to make it opaque, enabling Revlon to offer a much wider range of colours.

Bright-red nail varnish became the rage, especially when Wallis Simpson, the future Duchess of Windsor, took it up. Revson called one shade 'Wallis'; even then, he understood the importance of role models in selling cosmetics.

Later, he used famous beauties in Revlon's advertising campaigns. In the 1950s, it was flame-haired Suzy Parker, the super-model of her day.

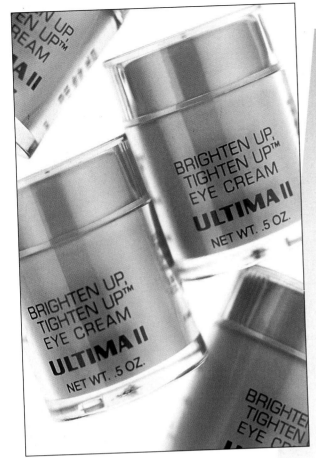

The 1960s' duo of gamine Twiggy and exotic Veruschka were followed in the 1970s and '80s by Lauren Hutton and Brooke Shields. More recently, Cindy Crawford and Claudia Schiffer have been Revlon models. Revlon set a modern trend by being the first to sign a model (Lauren Hutton) to an exclusive contract as the company's 'face'.

THE MAKE-UP BOOM

A Hollywood-influenced fashion for heavy make-up was well-entrenched in the 1930s and 1940s. The cosmetics industry was further stimulated by wartime scientific advances, such as the discoveries of lanolin and aerosols, as well as by increased prosperity following World War II.

Revlon was well to the fore with new or, some said, copycat products. Helena Rubinstein was convinced

that the company had stolen ideas for new skin treatments – *Skin Dew* and *Ultima* – from her *Youth Dew* and *Ultra Feminine* ranges. *Ultima* became one of the most successful of all Revlon lines. Another was the 'Co-ordinated Lip-and-Finger-Tip Makeup' – matching lipstick and nail varnish.

Clever promotion was important to Revlon's success. In the 1950s, Revson pioneered a new trend – away from ads stressing how a product could recapture youth towards a greater emphasis on

Above: Cindy Crawford was the 'face' of Revlon in the 1990s. Right: Revson named That Man *as a riposte to Elizabeth Arden. Helena Rubinstein thought that he copied her products, with* Ultima *(top left) derived from her* Ultra Feminine *range.*

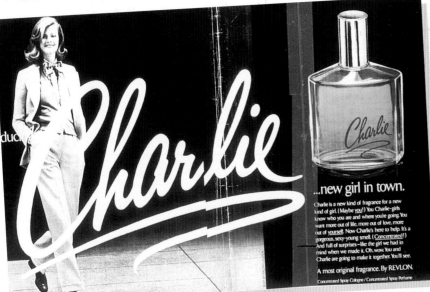

Charlie

...new girl in town.

Charlie is a new kind of fragrance for a new kind of girl. (Maybe you!) You Charlie-girls know who you are and where you're going. You want more out of life, more out of love, more out of yourself. Now Charlie's here to help. It's a gorgeous, sexy-young smell. (Concentrated!) And full of surprises—like the girl we had in mind when we made it. Oh, wow. You and Charlie are going to make it together. You'll see.

A most original fragrance. By REVLON.

Concentrated Spray Cologne / Concentrated Spray Perfume

Above: The early Charlie ad campaigns established the brand as a modern, youthful fragrance.
Left: Charlie Gold, like Charlie Red, is a pale amber liquid. Its shiny gold package, however, distinguishes it from its predecessor.

Revlon
C O L L E C T I O N

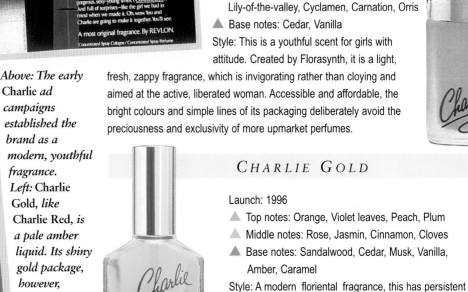

CHARLIE

Launch: 1973
▲ Top notes: Green notes, Citrus
▲ Middle notes: Jasmin, Rose, Lily-of-the-valley, Cyclamen, Carnation, Orris
▲ Base notes: Cedar, Vanilla

Style: This is a youthful scent for girls with attitude. Created by Florasynth, it is a light, fresh, zappy fragrance, which is invigorating rather than cloying and aimed at the active, liberated woman. Accessible and affordable, the bright colours and simple lines of its packaging deliberately avoid the preciousness and exclusivity of more upmarket perfumes.

CHARLIE GOLD

Launch: 1996
▲ Top notes: Orange, Violet leaves, Peach, Plum
▲ Middle notes: Rose, Jasmin, Cinnamon, Cloves
▲ Base notes: Sandalwood, Cedar, Musk, Vanilla, Amber, Caramel

Style: A modern floriental fragrance, this has persistent spicy elements mingling with rich, ripe fruit and the heady scents of midsummer flowers, finishing with the slight damp earthiness of musk and amber.

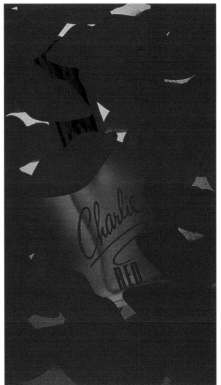

sexual allure. Revlon's deep red matching lipstick and nail polish, 'Fire and Ice', was sold under the slogans 'Are you made for Fire and Ice?' and 'There's a little bit of bad in every good woman'.

THE *CHARLIE* GIRL

A different style of advertising was used for the promotion of the mould-breaking perfume *Charlie*

Right: Charlie Red, released 20 years after the launch of the original, was the first variation on the Charlie formula.

(1973). Before *Charlie*, Revlon had launched a line of fragrances, with the sweet-chypre *Intimate* in 1955, followed by several more scents in the well-mannered, floral-oriental styles of the time. By contrast, *Charlie*, with its light, green-floral top notes and woody, vanilla undertones, was a totally new concept. It identified with liberated young women – feisty, self-confident, sexy, competitive and independent. The advertising reflected this. Misty, soft-focus romanticism was replaced by an energetic, youthful woman in a

CHARLIE SUNSHINE

Launch: 1997
- ▲ Top notes: Bergamot, Lemon, Mandarin, Pear, Fresh green notes
- ▲ Middle notes: Lily-of-the-valley, Freesia, Rose, Peony, Violet
- ▲ Base notes: Sandalwood, Amber, Musk

Style: *Charlie Sunshine* is just as fresh and youthful in its appeal as others in the *Charlie* range. It is designed as a light, sunny, summery fragrance which can be used all year round. The citrus top notes give it a zest and sparkle, and the sunny cheerfulness continues in the floral middle notes of muguet, freesia and rose, which are underpinned by a woody, musk base.

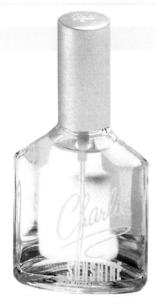

Left and right: Ads for the latest additions to the Charlie *range continue the uninhibited, youthful theme.*

CHARLIE SILVER

Launch: 1998
- ▲ Top notes: Pear, Vine flower
- ▲ Middle notes: Heather, Magnolia, Lily-of-the-valley, Lime-tree sap
- ▲ Base notes: Musk, Amber, Precious woods

Style: A fresh-fruity, floral eau de toilette, with crisp green notes on a clean, woody, musk base, this perfectly expresses 1990s cool with some interesting unorthodox accents. Fresh and uplifting, it is ideal for wearing on long, languid summer days.

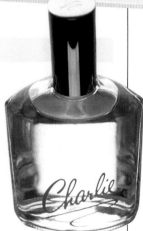

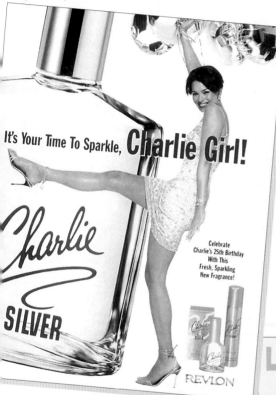

tweedy trouser suit, boots and jaunty beret, and the slogan 'The world belongs to Charlie'. It was an instant hit; *Charlie* became as much a part of every 1970s' teenager's wardrobe as platform shoes and bell-bottomed trousers.

In the 1990s, it is still going strong as *Charlie Red, White, Gold, Sunshine* and *Silver*, with fresh notes adapted to the changing mood of the times.

PROFILE

Revlon

1906 Charles Revson (below right) born in the USA.
1932 Founds Revlon with his brother, Joseph, and Charles Lachman.
1952 Launch of 'Fire and Ice' – matching lipstick and nail varnish – with innovatively sexual advertising campaign.
1955 Launch of first fragrance *Intimate*.
1973 Launch of *Charlie*.
1974 Lauren Hutton signed to pioneering exclusive contract.
1976 Charles Revson dies.
1985 Revlon bought by Ronald Perelman.

PERFUME CHRONOLOGY

1955	*Intimate*	**1975**	*Chaz*	**1994**	*Fire and Ice*
1961	*That Man*	**1980**	*Scoundrel*	**1994**	*Fire and Ice for Men*
1966	*Braggi*	**1980**	*Novell 2*		
1967	*Ultima 2*	**1988**	*Xia Xiang*	**1996**	*Charlie White*
1969	*Novell*	**1990**	*Unforgettable*	**1996**	*Charlie Blue*
1970	*Moon Drops*	**1993**	*Wild Heart*	**1996**	*Charlie Gold*
1973	*Charlie*	**1993**	*Charlie Red*	**1997**	*Charlie Sunshine*
1974	*Cerissa*	**1994**	*Ajee*	**1998**	*Charlie Silver*

SHISEIDO

In the century and more of its existence, Shiseido has grown from a Tokyo pharmacy to an international cosmetics and fragrance house that combines the best of East and West.

Yushin Fukuhara, a former chemist with the Japanese Navy, founded Shiseido as a Western-style pharmacy in Tokyo's fashionable shopping street of Ginza in 1872. The company philosophy then and now was to fuse tradition with technology, and oriental restraint and refinement with science and European flair.

Right: Shiseido's enigmatic graphic style was introduced by Artistic Director Serge Lutens. Below left: De Luxe was launched in Japan in 1945.

EAU ROUGE

The company, whose name is taken from a passage in the *I Ching* celebrating the beauties of the Earth, concentrated at first on pharmaceutical products, then launched into cosmetics with *Eudermine*. This innovative rose-

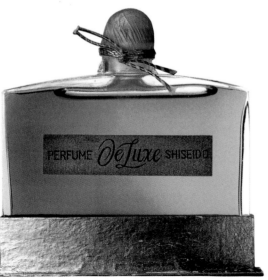

scented skin freshener and toning lotion – popular, it was rumoured, with geishas from the nearby Shimbashi district – was said to give the skin an incomparable texture and brightness. It came to be known as 'eau rouge' because of its brilliant magenta colour, and has recently been reformulated and relaunched. Coloured skin-tone face powder was another first, replacing the traditional Japanese chalk white.

Following an exhilarating trip to the Great Exhibition in Paris in 1900, Yushin's attraction to the

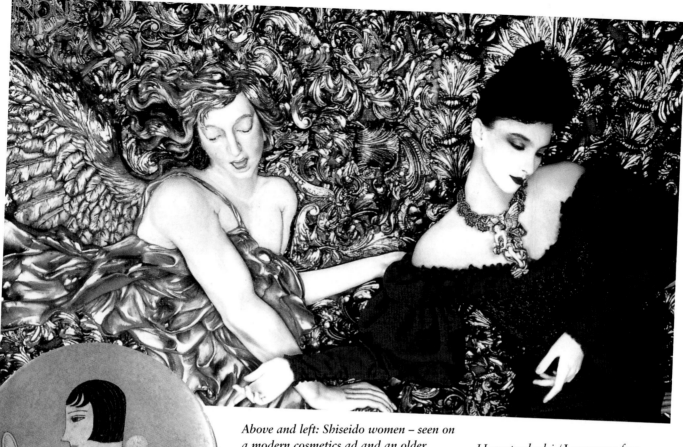

Above and left: Shiseido women – seen on a modern cosmetics ad and an older powder compact – combine images of East and West, often bearing the pale skin and red lips of a geisha.

Tokyo. He gathered a team of gifted young artists in the Shiseido Design Department to design ads, posters and packaging to the highest creative and production standards, establishing a Shiseido tradition that still continues.

One of Shinzo's designs was the camellia trademark which is still in use. With its sinuous lines and stylized shapes typical of Art Deco, it decorated Shiseido's first perfume

Right: Despite the success of its fragrances, the core business at Shiseido has always been cosmetics and toiletries, such as these in the Benefiance and Bio-Performance ranges.

Hanatsubaki (Japanese for 'camellia') in 1916.

Before then, perfumes made in Japan tended to imitate Western ones, but Shinzo tried to capture the essence of traditional Japanese flowers in his fragrances – wisteria, chrysanthemum, camellia, magnolia and plum blossom – producing new hybrids combining Western and oriental virtues. European styles were then chic

West became a full-blown love affair. In 1908, he sent his son Shinzo to Columbia University in New York. Afterwards, the young man spent a year in Paris imbibing French culture, meeting artists and musicians, and becoming a talented photographer.

NEW APPROACH

Shinzo's Parisian experience and the impact of Art Nouveau and, later, Art Deco, inspired him to introduce an ambitious, totally new approach to product design and advertising on his return to

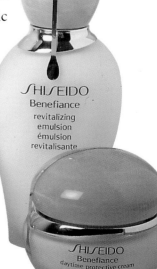

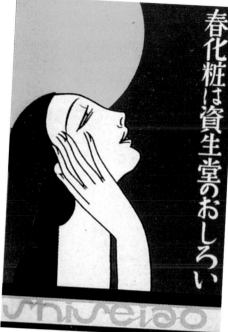

in Japan, and the packaging featured Lalique-style crystal bottles, Roman script and Western names.

The reverse was true of *Zen*, Shiseido's first perfume launched overseas in 1965. The Tokyo Olympics in 1964 had helped make Japanese style fashionable in the West, and the black and gold carton and flaçon were inspired by motifs in a Kyoto temple.

When the French photographer, designer and cosmetic artist Serge Lutens joined Shiseido as Creative Director in 1980, he, too, was deeply influenced by Japanese aesthetics. His work at Dior and on *Vogue* had been experimental – he was the first to introduce pink and yellow into eye colours. At Shiseido, he was given a free hand to create the company's international imagery.

Lutens created a series of striking advertising images for Shiseido, as well as devising their make-up colours and styles. He also conceived fragrances, such as

Above: Shiseido's Design Department has always used fine graphic artists to create images such as this one of 1926.

Féminité du Bois (1992), inspired by the scent of cedar in the Atlas Mountains of Morocco where he lives for half the year.

INNOVATORS

Shiseido's tradition of visual artistry has always been allied to technical know-how. Its Research Centre, founded in 1939, is unrivalled in the cosmetics industry. The company has pioneered the use of aromachology in fragrances, devising mood-altering perfumes that base herbal lore in solid scientific research. Creating fruitful alliances between the old and the new is still the Shiseido way.

Right: Exclusive scents developed by Lutens are on sale in the Salons du Palais Royal in Paris, or via the Internet.

PROFILE

Shiseido

1872 Founded by Yushin Fukuhara as a Western-style pharmacy in Ginza, Tokyo.
1897 Shiseido begins making cosmetics; introduces *Eudermine* skin toning lotion, the famous 'eau rouge'.
1908 Yushin's son Shinzo goes to New York to study pharmacology.
1916 Shiseido introduces its first perfume *Hanatsubaki*. Opens cosmetics shop in Tokyo. Shinzo establishes the Shiseido Design Department; designs the camellia (*hanatsubaki*) trademark.
1923 Launches network of chainstores that eventually cover Japan.
1927 Becomes a joint-stock company.
1937 Establishes the Camellia Club for customers, with monthly magazine.
1957 Begins expansion overseas.
1965 Establishes Shiseido Cosmetics America; launches *Zen* perfume – first product for overseas markets.
1980 Serge Lutens (below) joins Shiseido as Creative Director.
1986 Launches international salon network with French company Carita, now part of Shiseido group.
1990 Establishes Beauté Prestige International in Paris to direct fragrance business worldwide; creates couturier fragrances *Issey Miyake* (1992) and *Jean Paul Gaultier* (1993).
1991 Establishes first European factory at Gien, France.
1992 Opens the Salons du Palais Royal Shiseido in Paris.
1997 Relaunches *Eudermine*.

PERFUME CHRONOLOGY

1916 *Hanatsubaki*	**1981** *Nombre Noir*
1945 *De Luxe*	**1987** *Saso*
1964 *Zen* (first perfume issued outside Japan)	**1992** *Chant du Coeur, Lordes Neues, Blue Rose, Féminité du Bois*
1976 *Suzuro*	**1993** *Vivace, Basala*
1977 *Sourine*	**1997** *Relaxing Fragrance*
1978 *Tactics, Auslese, Mai*	**1998** *Vocalise*
1980 *Murasaki*	

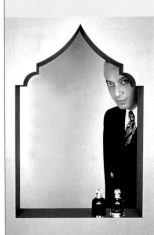

Shiseido

C O L L E C T I O N

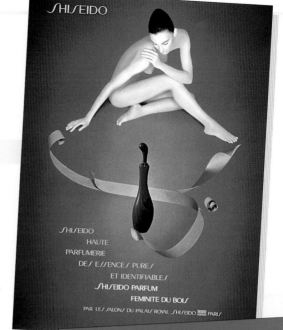

FÉMINITÉ DU BOIS

Launch: 1992

Dominant note: Cedarwood of Atlas Mountains

▲ Top notes: Neroli, Turkish rose

▲ Middle notes: Peach, Honey, Violet

▲ Base notes: Cardamom, Cinnamon, Clove, Musk, Vanilla

Style: Serge Lutens conceived this fragrance with an original structure based on a pure note of Moroccan cedarwood from the Atlas Mountains, which the other elements are chosen to enhance. The satiny warmth of the cedar core is deeply sensual and feminine and, heightened by fruity floral notes and hints of spice, is distinctive and alluring. The sinuous fla on symbolizes the female body in silent repose.

RELAXING FRAGRANCE

Launch: 1997

▲ Top notes: Artemisia, Young bamboo, Cucumber, Tea rose

▲ Middle notes: Peony, Gardenia, Cardamom

▲ Base notes: Sandalwood, Patchouli, Myrrh

Style: This wonderfully calming perfume in its cool, green, frosted bottle is inspired by state-of-the-art aromachological science backed by traditional herbal therapy. It aims to produce a sense of tranquillity, well-being and inner harmony. The floral-green-spicy notes restore balance, and sandalwood has been known for centuries for its ability to soothe the soul , while the stress-reducing effects of tea rose were the subject of rigorous testing by Shiseido.

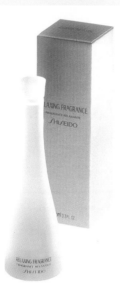

Right: The advertising style for all Shiseido fragrances concentrates on the expressive individual designs of each bottle, and combines them with background colour washes and a graphic style appropriate to the emotional quality or mood of the product.

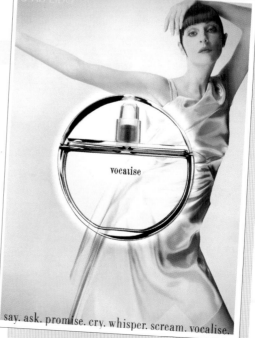

VOCALISE

Launch: 1998

▲ Notes: White orchid, Vanilla, Cassis, Yuzu, Pepper, Rose, Neroli, Lily-of-the-valley, Peach, Musk, Hinoki wood

Style: Created by top perfumer Jacques Cavallier, this sparkling fragrance is an entirely new type which breaks away from the traditional hierarchy of notes. The heady sweetness of white orchid is surrounded by fresh, floral-fruity scents, mingled with the intoxicating warmth of peaches, vanilla and musk, and the enticing oriental accents of Japanese hinoki wood.

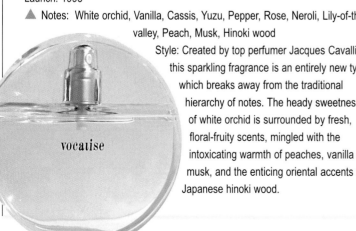

BALENCIAGA

The great Spanish couturier Balenciaga once described a fashion designer's existence as 'a dog's life', yet few were as dedicated, disciplined and passionate about their work as he was.

Above: Balenciaga's extraordinary feel for cloth, and his legendary tailoring skills allowed him to create some of the most extraordinary of all couture garments. This swirling gown dates from 1967.

Cristóbal Balenciaga Eisaguirre had a talent that took him from the tiny Basque fishing village where he was born to the peak of Paris fashion. He was enormously successful by any standards. In his heyday, from the 1940s to the 1960s, his clothes were on every wealthy woman's shopping list. His clients included Marlene Dietrich, Pauline de Rothschild, Princess Grace of Monaco and the queens of Belgium and Spain. He was universally respected and admired by other designers, and the originality and brilliance of his ideas and the sheer perfection of their execution left everyone else standing, including Dior. He was also a mentor to future stars, such as Givenchy, Oscar de la Renta, Courrèges and Ungaro.

Balenciaga's clothes were famously expensive. He refused to compromise on cut, fabric or ornamentation. As his dressmaker mother had taught him sewing and tailoring, he could do everything himself, unlike the majority of designers, and he involved himself in every detail, from cutting and stitching to making the buttonholes.

OUT OF THE LIMELIGHT

His rigorous attitude to his work was matched by an outwardly austere personality and a hidden private life. He was a loner, rarely photographed and almost never interviewed, who watched his own shows from behind a curtain. To those who knew him well, however, he was witty, elegant and charming, if sometimes waspish.

Balenciaga's talents were evident from very early on. Encouraged by the Marquesa de Casas Torres, a local aristocrat, he opened his first couture workshop in San Sebastian when he was 16, and then salons in Madrid and Barcelona. During the Spanish Civil War, he moved to Paris, where financial backing from some large fabric

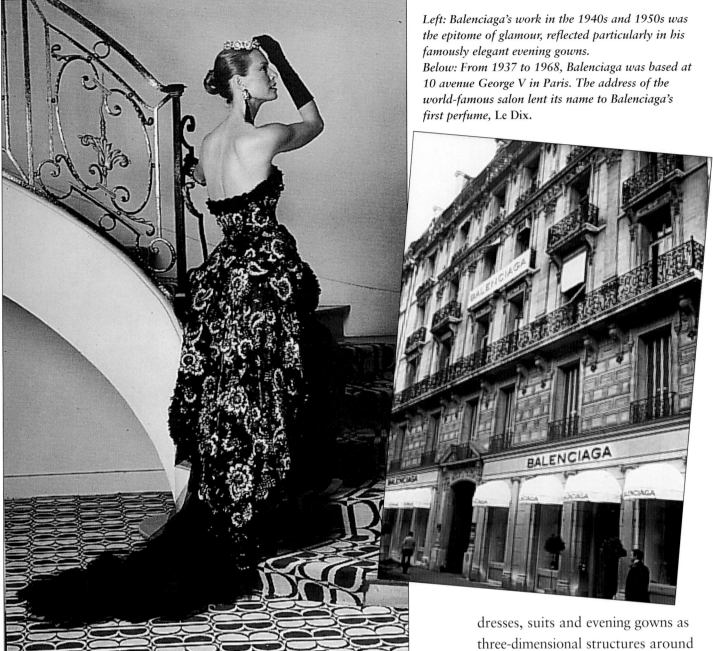

Left: Balenciaga's work in the 1940s and 1950s was the epitome of glamour, reflected particularly in his famously elegant evening gowns.
Below: From 1937 to 1968, Balenciaga was based at 10 avenue George V in Paris. The address of the world-famous salon lent its name to Balenciaga's first perfume, Le Dix.

manufacturers at last gave him a measure of financial stability. Balenciaga gowns figured large in the luxuries smuggled out of Paris after the German Occupation, but it was after the war that his great gifts at last reached fruition, and he was able to put into practice the ideas that made him unique.

'A couturier must be an architect for design,' he said, 'a sculptor for shape, a painter for colour, a musician for harmony, and a

philosopher for temperament.' He certainly had a genius for tailoring, and could create voluminous tent-like coats from single cloths with just a few tucks and darts.

THE GREAT INNOVATOR
He transformed the female silhouette by designing looser-fitting clothes that encircled rather than hugged the body, and were especially kind to women with less than perfect figures. He designed

dresses, suits and evening gowns as three-dimensional structures around the body rather than on it, and favoured fabrics, such as stiff silks and robust wools, that held their shape, and did not drift or drape.

He invented, among other things, the raised rollback collar that flatters the neckline, the three-quarter sleeve and the harem skirt, as well as the famous 'sack' dress, a shift dropping straight from wide shoulders to a narrow hem.

Balenciaga was a purist. Ready-to-wear garments never interested him, and he retired and closed his salons in 1968, rather than meet what he saw as crass, market-driven demands. He died in 1972.

The fashion company reopened in 1988 under new management, but in the same meticulous spirit. The house has a new chief designer in the shape of young Nicolas Guesquière, whose 1999 collection was much acclaimed.

When Balenciaga retired in 1968, he kept and maintained the perfume side of his business. His earliest perfume, *Le Dix*, brought him financial

Right: Balenciaga's third fragrance Ho Hang – the last released in his lifetime – is packaged in his favourite colours, red and black.

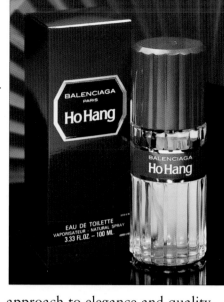

security for the first time. The name was taken from the address of his famous Paris salon, 10 avenue George V. Like his clothes, it was classic in conception.

EXPANDING RANGE

Quadrille and *Ho Hang* – the latter a fresh, unisex eau de toilette – were released in his lifetime, while *Michelle*, launched in memory of Balenciaga, was named after his favourite mannequin. Balenciaga expected the same rigorous

approach to elegance and quality to be applied to fragrance as to clothes. For him, perfume was simply 'fashion breathing all around us'. The fragrances produced after his death carried on this tradition.

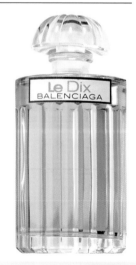

Balenciaga
C O L L E C T I O N

Left: The ads used to promote Le Dix and Rumba rely on pack shots and the Balenciaga name and logo to make their point. Extravagant promises – indeed, any words at all – are conspicuously absent.

LE DIX

Launch: 1947

▲ Top notes: Aldehydes, Bergamot, Lemon, Coriander, Peach

▲ Middle notes: Rose, Lily-of-the-valley, Jasmin, Ylang-ylang

▲ Base notes: Orris, Sandalwood, Vetiver, Civet, Musk, Vanilla

Style: A classic aldehydic floral fragrance, *Le Dix* expresses the key Balenciaga principles of restraint, balance and refinement, yet is also intensely romantic and feminine. The cool, lightly spicy top notes are enveloped by a richly sensuous core of exotic flowery scents, underpinned by precious woods and the timeless potency of musk and orris root. The name (meaning the ten) is taken from 10 avenue George V in Paris, the address of Balenciaga s famous salon.

RUMBA

Launch: 1988

▲ Top notes: Plum, Peach, Bergamot, Basil

▲ Middle notes: Tuberose, Jasmin, Rose, Orchid, Heliotrope, Magnolia, Gardenia, French marigold

▲ Base notes: Patchouli, Amber, Cypress, Cistus, Leather, Labdanum, Vanilla

Style: As the name, that of a lively Cuban dance, suggests, this chypre fragrance, with sweet, powdery undertones, is full of verve and vitality — a blend of Parisian sophistication with Latin American energy and sensuality. The ribbed, ovoid shape of the bottle was inspired by the form of the percussive rattle which gives the rumba its vivacious rhythm.

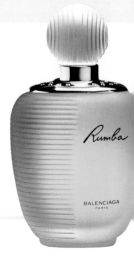

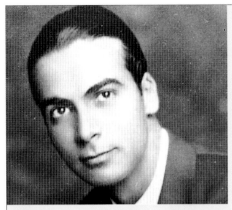

Balenciaga

PROFILE

1895 Cristóbal Balenciaga Eisaguirre (left) born in Guetaria, Spain.
1911 Starts a couture workshop in San Sebastian.
1915 Opens first salon in San Sebastian under his own name.
1920 Opens salons in Madrid and Barcelona.
1937 Opens the House of Balenciaga in Paris at 10 avenue George V.
1944 Introduces close-fitting waists and square shoulders.
1947 Launches first perfume, *Le Dix*.
1951 Introduces open necks, wide shoulders and looser waistlines.
1956 Invents the sack dress.
1958 Is awarded the Légion d'Honneur.
1968 Retires, closing salons in Paris, Barcelona and Madrid.
1972 Dies on 24 March in Valencia.
1988 Balenciaga Couture et Parfums acquired by Jacques and Régine Konckier; Michel Goma designs first collection.
1988 Balenciaga stores restyled by top designer Andrée Putman.
1993 Josephus Melchior Thimister becomes chief designer.
1998 Nicolas Guesquière takes over as chief designer.

PERFUME CHRONOLOGY

1947 *Le Dix*	**1980** *Michelle*
1955 *Quadrille*	**1982** *Prélude*
1971 *Ho Hang*	**1988** *Rumba*
1973 *Cialenga*	**1990** *Balenciaga*
1973 *Eau de*	*pour Homme*
Balenciaga	**1996** *Talisman*
Lavande	**1999** *Cristóbal*

TALISMAN

Launch: 1996

▲ Top notes: Blackcurrant, Bergamot, Violet leaf, Lychee, Indian artemisia (davana), Osmanthus, Dried fruits, Rum, Mandarin, Grapefruit

▲ Middle notes: Clove, Lily-of-the-valley, Freesia, Rose, Jasmin, Hyacinth, Orchid, Ylang-ylang, Cyclamen

▲ Base notes: Patchouli, Sandalwood, Oakmoss, Benzoin, Amber, Labdanum, Styrax, Vanilla, Beeswax

Style: This oriental chypre-style fragrance is a vibrant exotic blend of fruits, spices and tropical flowers, combining classical inspiration with resolutely modern intentions. Seductive, but in a light-hearted way, the fragrance is presented in an amphora-shaped flacon with Egyptian styling. The sunshine yellow carton is embellished with a graphic symbol that suggests both an ancient runic sign and the couturier's needle and thread.

Right: Befitting their more oriental, spicy nature, both Talisman *and* Cristóbal *are advertised with sexual imagery reflecting the shape of* Talisman's *bottle and the amber colour of* Cristóbal.

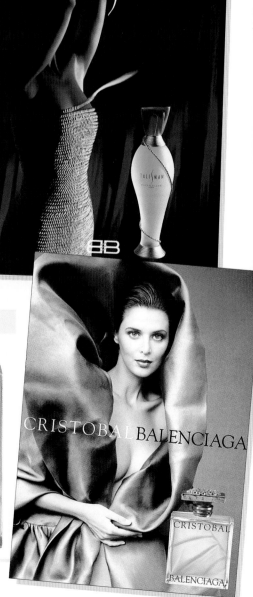

CRISTÓBAL

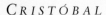

Launch: 1999

▲ Top notes: Fig leaves, Bergamot, Marigold

▲ Middle notes: Jasmin, Blue freesia, Peony

▲ Base notes: Sandalwood, Patchouli, Vanilla

Style: An intoxicating, oriental-style fragrance, *Cristóbal* evokes both cool, classical elegance and a more overt modern sensuality. It has stimulating, fresh top notes, with gentle, soft floral elements at the heart, all underscored by luxurious warm sandalwood and vibrant vanilla. Its advertising promotes a luminous image of eternal femininity in the form of a beautiful woman, whose billowing hooded cloak recalls the voluminous shapes of Balenciaga's famous coats and evening gowns. The ornate gold stopper of the square-shaped bottle hints at his taste for richly baroque embroidery and beading.

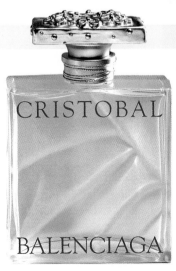

ROCHAS

Marcel Rochas made an indelible mark on the world of couture and perfumery in his relatively short life. After his death, his glamorous young widow took the company on to new levels of success.

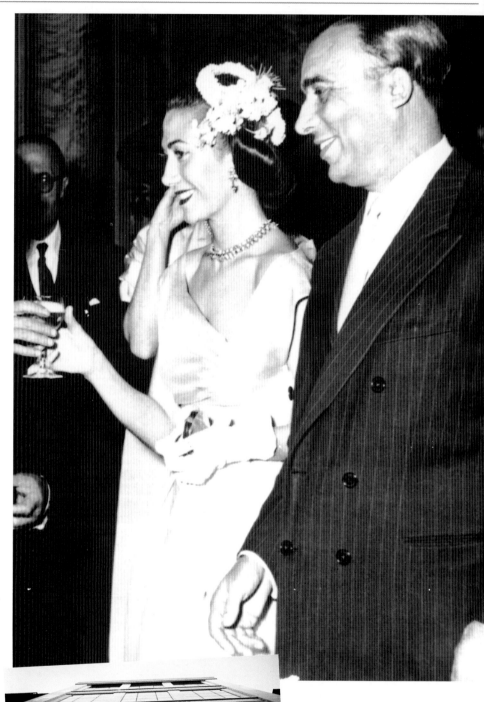

Born in Paris in 1902 and trained as a lawyer, Marcel Rochas became a fashion designer almost by accident, in order to supply the expensive tastes of his young wife, a former model. Rochas was an immensely creative designer and a shrewd businessman in equal measures. A stream of innovations drove his success.

ELEGANT INNOVATOR

His clothes were elegant, youthful and, above all, very feminine – even the slacks that he introduced for daywear in the early 1930s. With Schiaparelli, he invented the classic, broad-shouldered silhouette of the 1930s. He used fur imaginatively, treating it with bright dyes, and loved adventurous materials, such as animal-skin prints, flexible 'knit' fabrics and shiny metallics. Wide, white collars framing the face and plunging bare-back necklines were other Rochas trademarks.

Above: The course of Marcel Rochas's career was bound up with his wives; he entered the couture business to please his first wife, while Hélène, his second wife (above), was the inspiration for several perfumes. Left: Rochas's Paris headquarters are near the Champs-Elysées.

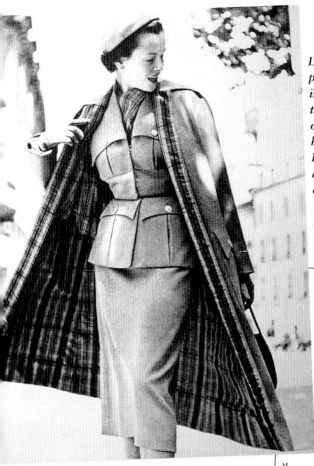

Left: Rochas sold exclusive perfumes in his couture house in 1936, but discontinued them in 1940 when the occupation of Paris cut off his supply of raw materials He continued to design clothes, however, such as this ensemble of 1940.

Below: Designs by Peter O'Brien revivified Rochas's couture house in the 1990s.

Marcel launched three exclusive perfumes, sold only at his salon in Avenue Matignon, in 1936, but *Femme* – dedicated to his second wife, Hélène – was the first to be launched by Parfums Rochas, founded in 1944. The voluptuously curved bottle was used for three more fragrances, with different-coloured lace on the box:

His flattering, often flamboyant styles found favour with film stars, such as Carole Lombard, Marlene Dietrich and Jean Harlow. Rochas, who appreciated the pulling power of Hollywood, courted them assiduously on his regular visits to California; he designed costumes for many films.

THE WASPIE

Mae West was a particular friend and inspired his most famous invention, the 'waspie' – a long-line strapless bra and corset combined – trimmed with her favourite black Chantilly lace. It made possible the hour-glass silhouette of the late 1940s, anticipating Dior's New Look. The black lace became the signature packaging of Rochas's most famous perfume *Femme*, an intensely seductive fragrance.

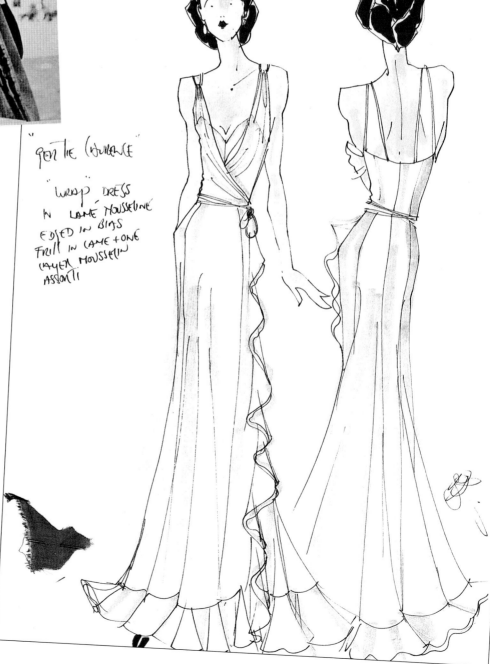

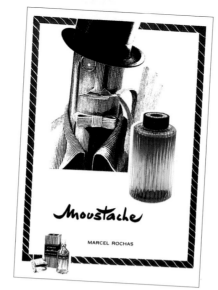

Right: The launch of Moustache *in 1949 represented the first-ever complete line of fragrance products for men.*

Mousseline in gold lace, *Mouche* – named after Marcel's cat – in turquoise and *La Rose* in pink.

HÉLÈNE AT THE HELM

Marcel died young in 1955, after closing the couture house to focus on perfumes and accessories. Hélène, just 28, became the youngest-ever head of a major perfume company. Five years later she produced *Madame Rochas*, a fragrance very much in her own image. With *Eau de Rochas* and *Mystère*, it made Rochas again a top name in perfume in the 1960s.

Hélène withdrew from the company in the late 1970s but was creative consultant on *Byzance*. The latest phase in the Rochas story has continued the innovative flair of its founder, with fragrances such as *Tocade*, *Alchimie* and *Rochas Man*, and mimicked his astute commercial instincts in the relaunch of *Femme* and *Madame Rochas*.

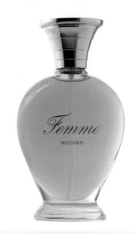

Rochas
COLLECTION

FEMME

Launch: 1945 (relaunched 1989)

▲ Top notes: Peach, Plum, Apricot, Bergamot, Cinnamon

▲ Middle notes: Jasmin, Rose, Everlasting flower Ylang-ylang

▲ Base notes: Oakmoss, Sandalwood, Musk, Am Patchouli, Vanilla

Style: The scent of the 1950s was created by Edm Roudnitska, Rochas s in-house perfumer. It is a cla fruity chypre with a distinctive, lusciously sweet pea top note, an intensely sensual flowery heart and ric woody-musky undertones. The bottle — modelled o Mae West s torso — was designed by Rochas and for several of his other fragrances. The black lace on the packaging became a defining icon of Rocha *Femme* was relaunched in 1989 for a younger clientele, with a new, fresher, lighter and spicier form

Below: The advertising for Femme's *relaune went for an earthy appeal. By contrast, ear ads featured a 'face' from a Botticelli paint*

PROFILE

Rochas

1900 Marcel Rochas born in Paris.

1925 Opens House of Rochas in rue Faubourg St Honoré in Paris.

1931 Moves to 12 avenue Matignon.

1943 Marries Hélène Rochas.

1944 Founds Parfums Rochas in partnership with Alfred Gosset.

1945 Launches *Femme*, his first perfume for the general market.

1946 Introduces the 'waspie' corset.

1953 Closes couture house to concentrate on perfumes and accessories.

1955 Marcel dies; Hélène Rochas becomes president.

1970 Hélène Rochas steps down as president, leaving Gosset in charge.

1975 Gosset retires; Rochas acquired by Roussel-Uclaf.

1987 German cosmetics group Wella buys Rochas; *Femme* relaunched.

1989 *Madame Rochas* relaunched; Hélène Rochas retires.

1990 Reintroduction of ready-to-wear collections, with Peter O'Brien (left) as chief designer.

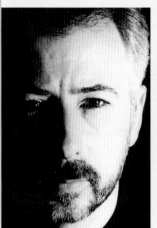

PERFUME CHRONOLOGY

1945 *Femme*	**1970** *Eau de Rochas*
1947 *Mousseline*	**1978** *Mystère*
1948 *Eau de Verveine*	**1984** *Lumière*
1948 *Eau de Roche*	**1987** *Byzance*
1948 *Mouche*	**1994** *Tocade*
1949 *La Rose*	**1995** *Byzantine*
1949 *Moustache*	**1996** *Fleur d'Eau*
1960 *Madame Rochas*	**1997** *Tocadilly*
1969 *Monsieur Rochas*	**1998** *Alchimie*

FEMME. TRÈS FEMME.

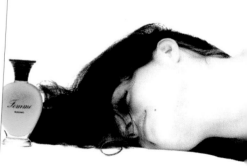

ROCHAS

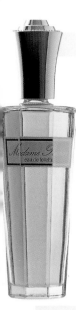

MADAME ROCHAS

Launch: 1960 (relaunched 1989)

▲ Top notes: Neroli, Broom, Honeysuckle

▲ Middle notes: Ylang-ylang, Tuberose, Jasmin, Orris, Bulgarian rose, Lilac, Lily-of-the-valley, Orange blossom

▲ Base notes: Sandalwood, Cedar, Musk, Amber, Vetiver

Style: *Madame Rochas*, a classic, soft, floral scent created by Guy Robert, has around 200 ingredients. It has a cooler, more delicate appeal than *Femme*, and evokes grace, elegance and a refined glamour rather than sensuality. Fresh, gentle top notes dissolve into a soft, powdery, floral centre with rose and lily-of-the-valley accents. The octagonal fla on, inspired by an antique smelling-salts bottle in the collection of H l ne Rochas — again the inspiration for the fragrance — was Pierre Dinand s first perfume bottle design. An 18th-century tapestry design was used on the box. The fragrance was updated with a slightly more intensified formula in 1989.

BYZANCE

Launch: 1987

▲ Top notes: Citrus, Cardamom, Aldehydes

▲ Middle notes: Rose, Jasmin, Tuberose, Orris, Lily-of-the-valley

▲ Base notes: Sandalwood, Musk, Vanilla, Amber, Heliotrope, Patchouli

Style: Created by Nicholas Mamounas, Rochas s in-house perfumer in the 1970s and 1980s, this floral-oriental fragrance skilfully blends eastern and western elements into a complex, subtle and harmonious brew that manages to combine elegance, sensuality, coolness and exoticism. Fresh aldehydic top notes give way to a spicy, floral heart, followed by the warm intensity of richly scented heliotrope, musk and vanilla. The blue bottle reflects Rochas house colours and the tones of Byzantine mosaics.

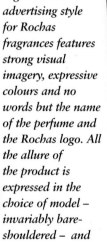

Right: The house advertising style for Rochas fragrances features strong visual imagery, expressive colours and no words but the name of the perfume and the Rochas logo. All the allure of the product is expressed in the choice of model – invariably bare-shouldered – and the setting.

ALCHIMIE

Launch: 1998

▲ Top notes: Blackcurrant, Bergamot, Grapefruit

▲ Middle notes: Jasmin, Acacia, Passion flower

▲ Base notes: Vanilla, Sandalwood, Tonka bean

Style: Introducing a new olfactory family, the fresh floral-sensual, this elegant but accessible modern perfume fuses Rochas s traditional image of refined French luxury and sophistication with a more contemporary approach aimed at the international marketplace. It offers an enticing blend of blackcurrant with the fruity sparkle of grapefruit and bergamot and the voluptuous warmth of vanilla and sandalwood. Soft, velvety floral notes form the heart. The bottle, designed by Serge Mansau, expresses Marcel Rochas s classic watchwords — elegance, youth and simplicity.

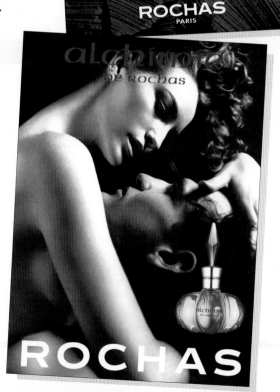

BALMAIN

Pierre Balmain, one of the creators of the post-war New Look, with its fitted bodices and full skirts, was noted for his cool, elegant styles. He also created several celebrated fragrances, hailed today as perfume classics.

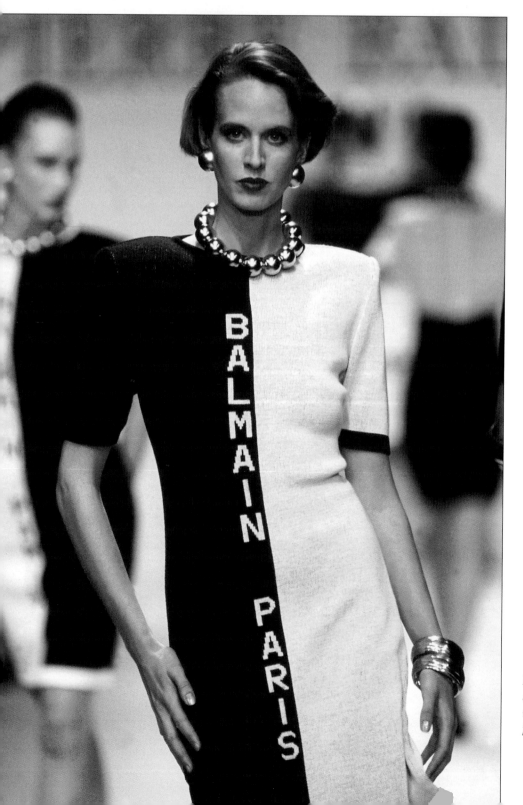

When Pierre Balmain left his native Savoie in 1933 to study architecture at the École des Beaux-Arts in Paris, he took with him letters of introduction to several leading couturiers. As a student, he scribbled ideas for gowns, coats and hats in the margins of his architectural blueprints, just as in later years he sketched windows, parapets and cornices on fashion drawings. In 1934, though, Balmain sold some sketches to couturier Robert Piguet, and his career choice was made.

RESTRAINED STYLE

Balmain brought a modernist architectural sensibility to his creations. His style was classical with pure, simple lines – he created cool elegance with tremendous grace and poise. Understatement was his trademark and he abhorred what he considered vulgar display and ostentatious ornament. His colours were typically soft or sober – lemon yellow, ice blue, pale lilac, mint green, navy, maroon or charcoal grey. The daytime silhouette was

Left: Under the American designer Oscar de la Renta, Balmain haute couture retained the simple, elegant lines made famous by Balmain himself.

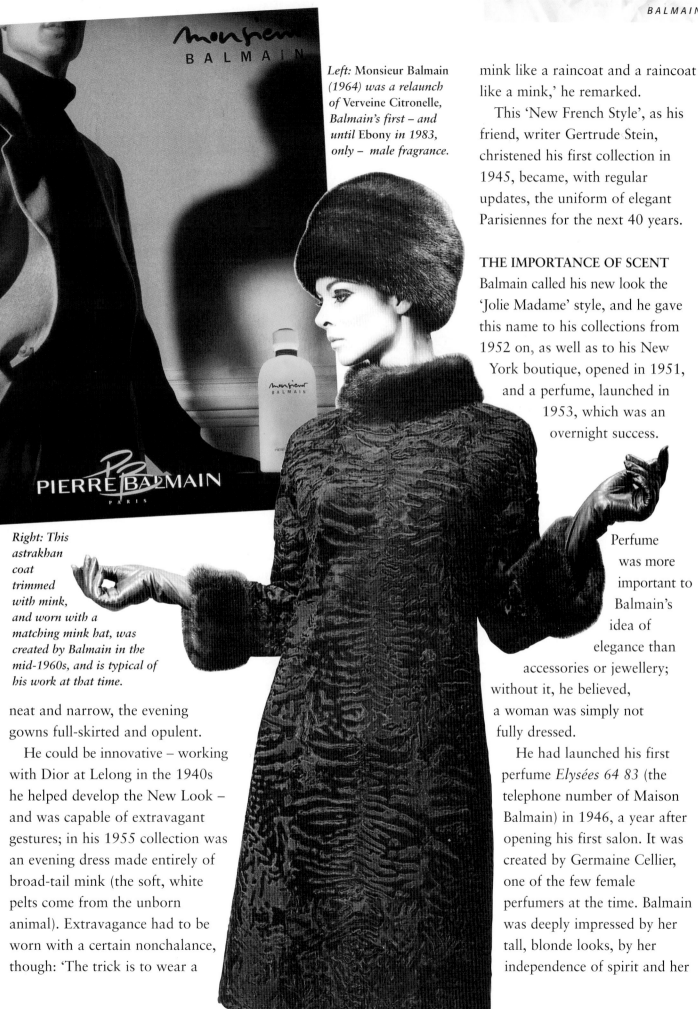

Left: Monsieur Balmain *(1964) was a relaunch of* Verveine Citronelle, *Balmain's first – and until* Ebony *in 1983, only – male fragrance.*

PIERRE BALMAIN
PARIS

Right: This astrakhan coat trimmed with mink, and worn with a matching mink hat, was created by Balmain in the mid-1960s, and is typical of his work at that time.

neat and narrow, the evening gowns full-skirted and opulent.

He could be innovative – working with Dior at Lelong in the 1940s he helped develop the New Look – and was capable of extravagant gestures; in his 1955 collection was an evening dress made entirely of broad-tail mink (the soft, white pelts come from the unborn animal). Extravagance had to be worn with a certain nonchalance, though: 'The trick is to wear a

mink like a raincoat and a raincoat like a mink,' he remarked.

This 'New French Style', as his friend, writer Gertrude Stein, christened his first collection in 1945, became, with regular updates, the uniform of elegant Parisiennes for the next 40 years.

THE IMPORTANCE OF SCENT
Balmain called his new look the 'Jolie Madame' style, and he gave this name to his collections from 1952 on, as well as to his New York boutique, opened in 1951, and a perfume, launched in 1953, which was an overnight success.

Perfume was more important to Balmain's idea of elegance than accessories or jewellery; without it, he believed, a woman was simply not fully dressed.

He had launched his first perfume *Elysées 64 83* (the telephone number of Maison Balmain) in 1946, a year after opening his first salon. It was created by Germaine Cellier, one of the few female perfumers at the time. Balmain was deeply impressed by her tall, blonde looks, by her independence of spirit and her

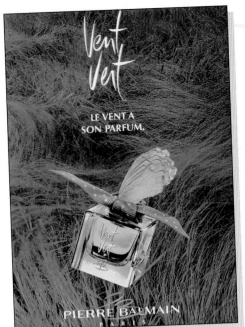

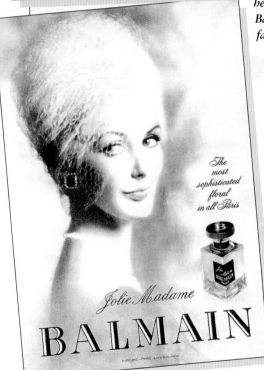

Balmain
COLLECTION

Left: The texts for the Vent Vert *and* Jolie Madame *ads – 'The breeze has its own scent' and 'The most sophisticated floral in all Paris' – both express the cool elegance at the heart of the Balmain fashion ethos.*

VENT VERT

Launch: 1945
▲ Top notes: Agrumen oils (citrus), Bergamot, Neroli, Violet leaf
▲ Middle notes: Basil, Galbanum, Lily-of-the-valley, Freesia, Rose, Hyacinth, Jasmin
▲ Base notes: Sage, Sandalwood, Oakmoss, Musk
Style: This innovative fragrance, the first green-floral scent in the history of perfumery, is essentially vivacious, full of energy and high spirits. It begins with a citrus freshness mingled with the soft delicacy of orange blossom and violets, followed by a heady bouquet of summer flowers tinged with the oily sharpness of basil and galbanum, and more serious sensual notes in sage and sandalwood. Its brisk, vibrant but lightly sensual qualities put it ahead of its time; it still smells like a modern perfume.

JOLIE MADAME

Launch: 1953
▲ Top notes: Lemon wood, Clove, Neroli, Gardenia, Artemisia
▲ Middle notes: Neroli, Violet leaf, Lilac, Jasmin, Tuberose, Orris
▲ Base notes: Oakmoss, Cedar, Patchouli, Castoreum
Style: A floral-oriental scent created by Germaine Cellier, this is totally evocative of the Balmain style — utterly elegant and sophisticated but with a dash of insolence. It has an intensely floral presence, rich yet fresh, which balances spice with delicacy and coolness with sensuality. The composition is tempered with leathery, mossy base notes.

creative ingenuity. In 1947 she came up with a landmark fragrance for Balmain. *Vent Vert* was a total breakthrough in perfumery, the first 'green' fragrance, with the exhilarating sappy freshness of damp woods after rain. It became the scent of choice for the liberated, sporty woman of the post-war period and spawned many imitators.

If *Vent Vert* refreshed the body, Cellier's next female fragrance, *Jolie Madame*, stirred the soul. With its potent violet note it was, in Balmain's words, a perfume 'for adventure, passion, enchantment'. It was an instant sensation and confirmed Balmain as a major international perfume house. A male companion fragrance, *Monsieur Balmain*, followed a decade later. *Miss Balmain* (1967) brought a new, more

youthful accent, perfectly in tune with the innocent 'little girl' suits that were his nod towards the 1960s' youth culture.

Balmain, who also designed for the theatre and films – producing wardrobes for Ava Gardner, Sophia Loren, Cyd Charisse and Bridget Bardot among others – died in 1982, leaving the company in

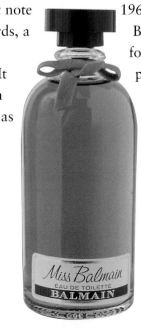

Left: Miss Balmain was launched in 1967, and was seen as a complement to the youthful styles of the day.

IVOIRE

Launch: 1979

▲ Top notes: Mandarin, Bergamot, Violet leaf

▲ Middle notes: Jasmin, Orris, Ylang-ylang, Rose, Lily-of-the-valley

▲ Base notes: Vetiver, Oakmoss, Sandalwood, Labdanum, Amber, Vanilla

Style: This is a classic green-floral fragrance with lasting undertones of precious woods and spices. It is exquisitely refined and elegant, a complex composition of enticing green top notes and voluptuous richness in its extravagantly floral heart, with warm vanilla and woody, amber base notes. It has a sultry, exotic quality, but one which is restrained by its essentially classy nature — an evening scent for adventurous sophisticates.

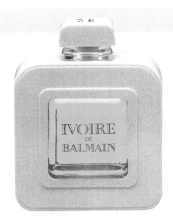

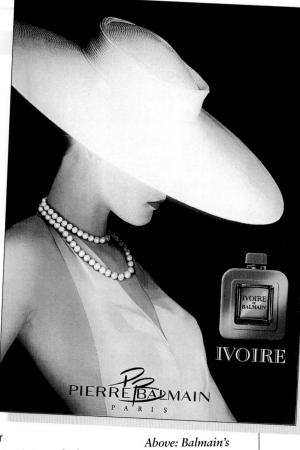

IVOIRE

PIERRE BALMAIN
PARIS

BALMAIN DE BALMAIN

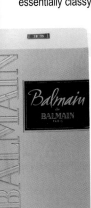

Launch: 1999

▲ Top notes: Bergamot, Galbanum, Black pepper, Blackcurrant

▲ Middle notes: Jasmin, Violet, Cabbage rose, Orris

▲ Base notes: Patchouli, Oakmoss, Sandalwood, Vetiver

Style: A green chypre fragrance characterized by the contrast between fresh, green, spicy top notes and a warm base, this has an immediate, radiant and happy appeal, full of *joie de vivre*, which is followed by a richer, more opulent and ultra-feminine floral core, and finished with a woody base. Its elegance is approachable and warm, rather than chilly. The simple modernist bottle, with its clean, sharp lines, was designed by Pierre Balmain himself in 1947 and updated by Xavier Rousseau.

Above: Balmain's love of hats – he once declared that 'women must not abdicate this weapon' – is reflected in the ads for Ivoire.

the hands of his right-hand man, Erik Mortensen. However, there were financial difficulties and it was sold and resold several times.

NEW ERA

Eventually Mortensen left, and an American, Oscar de la Renta, became artistic director. In 1998 the dynamic Giles DuFour was lured from Chanel to take over the ready-to-wear lines. His bright colours, short mini-skirts, jaunty feathers and glittering sequins threw off Balmain's decorous image and reinvented the house.

Balmain

1914 Pierre Balmain (below) born on 18 May in Savoie, France.

1933-4 Studies architecture at the École des Beaux-Arts, Paris.

1934 Becomes design assistant to Molyneux.

1945 Founds Maison Balmain in Paris.

1946 Launches first perfume *Elysées 64 83*.

1951 Opens salon in New York.

1952 First of the Jolie Madame collections.

1960 Perfume business bought by Revlon.

1978 Balmain awarded the Légion d'Honneur.

1982 Balmain dies; company resold.

1993 Oscar de la Renta becomes artistic director of couture collections.

1998 Giles DuFour heads ready-to-wear lines.

PERFUME CHRONOLOGY

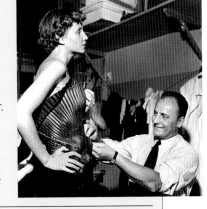

1946 *Elysées 64 83*	**1964** *Monsieur Balmain*	**1979** *Ivoire*
1947 *Vent Vert*	– a relaunch of	**1983** *Ebène*
1949 *Verveine Citronelle*	*Verveine Citronelle*	**1999** *Balmain de*
1953 *Jolie Madame*	**1967** *Miss Balmain*	*Balmain*

CACHAREL

The fresh, youthful appeal of Cacharel ready-to-wear lines has also been expressed in its fragrances, starting with the successful and groundbreaking Anaïs Anaïs in 1978.

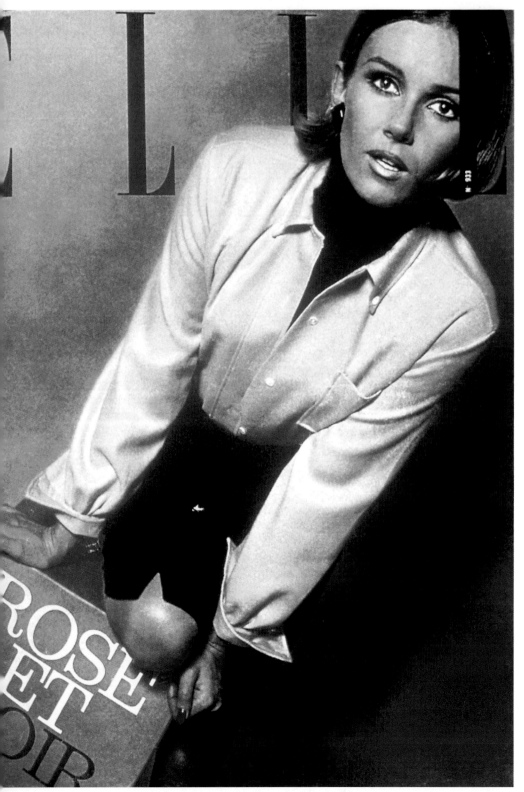

In 1962, Emmanuelle Kahn, a former Balenciaga and Givenchy model, announced that 'Haute couture is dead!' She was speaking as a stylist for the new Cacharel ready-to-wear company, created by designer Jean Bousquet. The explosion of 1960s' youth culture – when young women had neither the means nor the desire to buy the expensively tailored, one-off couture clothes coveted by their mothers – had created fertile ground for a new type of fashion company.

OFF-THE-PEG FASHION

The most exciting new designers – Kahn, Mary Quant, Biba Hulanicki and another Cacharel stylist, Agnès Troublé (later Agnès B) – ignored couture altogether. In a few years, ready-to-wear, formerly the poor relation of the fashion world, had triumphed; couturiers scuttled to open boutiques.

At the beginning of the 1960s, a *cacharel* simply meant a wild duck from the wetlands of the Camargue, near Bousquet's native

Left: An appearance on the front cover of Elle in 1963, promoting the crêpon blouse, propelled Cacharel to enormous success through the 1960s and '70s.

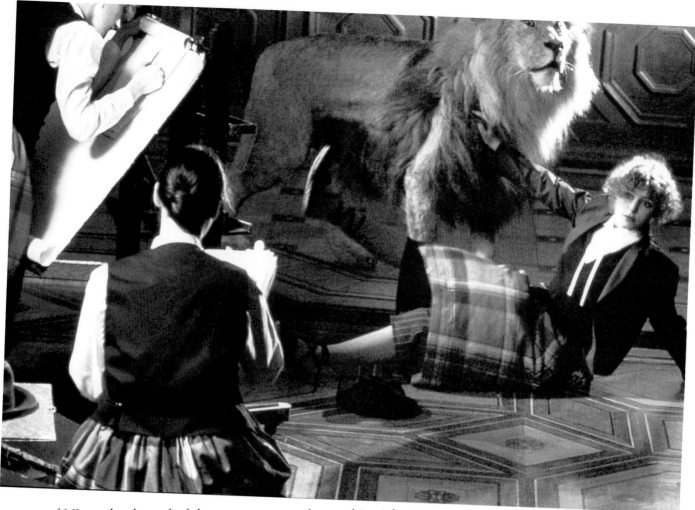

town of Nîmes; by the end of the decade, to the thousands of women who had a Cacharel hanging in their wardrobes, it meant a beautifully fitted, printed cotton shirt.

NEW IDEAS

Bousquet began in men's tailoring. He intended to join forces with his friend Charles Martin, but they disagreed about the name of the new company, among other things.

While Martin reinvented himself as Jacques Esterel, Bridget Bardot's favourite couturier, Bousquet became Jean Cacharel, king of ready-to-wear. The company, concentrating on separates, had a fresh, youthful, sporty image, free of the dull conventions. Designers experimented with cut (shirts with

narrow, almost skin-tight sleeves and no bust darts) and fabrics – the crêpon blouse, made from a featherweight crinkly cotton usually reserved for lingerie, was a runaway bestseller.

By the late 1960s, miniskirts, futuristic Paco Rabanne specs and spangles and cropped Vidal Sassoon haircuts had given way to the drifting frocks, ethnic beads and flowing tresses of the hippie generation. Cacharel tuned into the new spirit, and his first collection for men in 1968 featured the flowery shirts and

Above: The Cacharel style and appeal owes a great deal to the dreamy, soft-focus advertising imagery of photographer Sarah Moon.
Below: Loulou Blue, *launched in 1995, is a fresher, more delicate version of the seductive* Loulou.

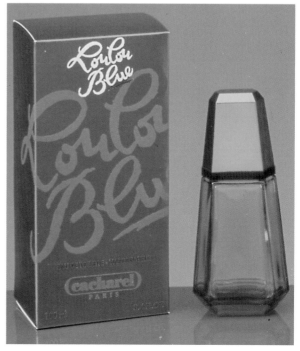

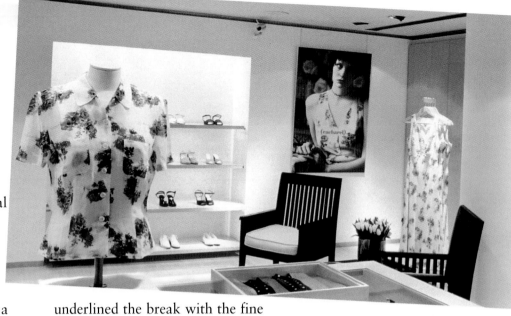

Right: The first exclusive Cacharel boutique in France opened in 1971. Now there are 40 worldwide.

velvet hipster pants which became the hippie uniform.

This mood of gentle romanticism, tinged with rural nostalgia, became the badge of Cacharel. It was this approach that appealed to L'Oréal when, in the mid-1970s, they were looking for a perfume with youthful appeal.

FIRST FRAGRANCE

Anaïs Anaïs (1978) was a groundbreaking scent. Named after a Persian goddess of fertility and death, it expressed a semi-mystical duality of light and dark, innocence and sensuality. Annegret Beier, who was to become Cacharel's regular flaçon designer,

underlined the break with the fine fragrance tradition with an innovative white opaline bottle.

A similarly enigmatic persona inspired *Loulou*, Cacharel's next female fragrance. She was again a goddess, but this time of the silver screen – the beautiful and wayward Louise Brooks, as seen in her role as Lulu in the 1929 classic *Pandora's Box*. Dangerously provocative, bewitching and

amoral, Lulu is also tender and naïve – the source of her fatal attraction. A wild, wilful sensuality is the keynote of the fragrance, provided principally by vanilla.

The link between innocence and temptation was explored again in *Eden* (1994), a luscious blend of sweet violet and orange blossom with enticing fruits, mimosa and patchouli. In *Loulou Blue* (1995), the mood is fresher and more delicate, while *Eau d'Eden* (1996) brings a lighter, crisper note to its exotic predecessor. Its aquatic notes, with scents of green leaves and wild flowers, are perhaps intended to recall the shimmering Camargue, whose free-flying water birds inspired Cacharel's ever-youthful image.

Right: The advertising style for Eau d'Eden *combines in a single image youthful playfulness, the idea of a paradisiacal flower garden and fresh cool water.*

PROFILE

Cacharel

1932 Jean Bousquet born in Nîmes, France.
1947 Bousquet apprenticed to a tailor.
1951 Becomes student at École Technique, Nîmes.
1956 Moves to Paris and works as cutter/stylist for Jean Jourdan.
1958 Opens studio making men's shirts.
1962 Bousquet (below, with models) founds Cacharel company making ready-to-wear clothes for women. Emmanuelle Khan joins as chief designer and stylist; introduction of famous crêpon blouses.
1966 Designer Corinne Sarrut (Bousquet's sister-in-law) joins Cacharel.
1967 Cacharel begins making men's shirts in Liberty prints.

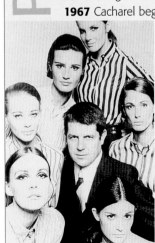

1968 Launches first collection for men.
1969 Launches children's collection.
1978 Launches first perfume *Anaïs Anaïs*.
1998 Launches new range of menswear shops and franchises, with shop-fitting and design by architect Norman Foster.

PERFUME CHRONOLOGY

1978 *Anaïs Anaïs*	**1994** *Eden*
1981 *Cacharel pour Homme*	**1995** *Loulou Blue*
	1996 *Eau d'Eden*
1987 *Loulou*	**1999** *Noa*

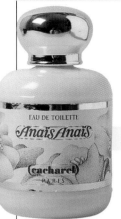

Cacharel
COLLECTION

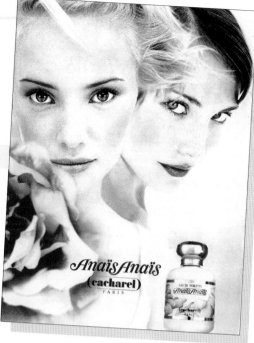

ANAÏS ANAÏS

Launch: 1978
- ▲ Top notes: Hyacinth, Orange blossom
- ▲ Middle notes: Tuberose, Jasmin, Honeysuckle, Lily-of-the-valley, Rose, Carnation, Ylang-ylang, Orris
- ▲ Base notes: Sandalwood, Cedar, Vetiver, Amber, Frankincense, Musk, Leather

Style: Designed to capture the mid-1970s youth market dedicated to natural fragrances and cosmetics, this is a light, floral perfume, soft and feminine, sweet and romantic, evoking purity and innocence. Created by Roger Pellegrino of Firmenich, it has a gently caressing, delicately floral heart, based on white flowers, with fresh, bright, leafy-green top notes and an ambery, musky finish. A truly youthful fragrance, appealing and affordable, it was an instant and huge success, much imitated in the 1980s.

Above: Anaïs Anaïs *has always had a very youthful image.*

LOULOU

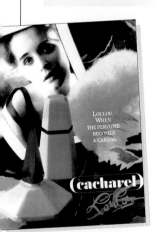

Launch: 1987
- ▲ Top notes: Bergamot, Blackcurrant buds, Green leaves, Marigold, Mandarin
- ▲ Middle notes: Jasmin, Heliotrope, Mimosa, Tiare flower, Ylang-ylang
- ▲ Base notes: Vanilla, Frankincense, Orris, Musk, Sandalwood, Tonka bean

Style: This oriental-floral perfume, created by Jean Guichard, is intoxicating, with sharp, lemony top notes merging into a bouquet of exotic blooms, including the bewitching tiare flowers of Tahiti, followed by a cascade of incense, tropical woods and spices. Annegret Beier s fla on with soaring red stopper was considered very avant-garde at the time.

Above: Loulou *is marketed as a sensual fragrance.*

EAU D'EDEN

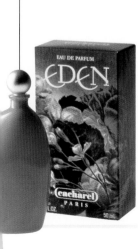

Launch: 1996
- ▲ Top notes: Flag iris, Hyacinth, Nasturtium
- ▲ Middle notes: Peach, Nectarine, Wild rose, Sweet William
- ▲ Base notes: Musk, Sandalwood

Style: A floral-fruity, musky fragrance, this is designed to evoke the crystal purity and sparkle of spring water, or the freshness of dewdrops on flower petals. Cool, tangy top notes of water iris, hyacinth and nasturtium, which suggest sunshine and light, are filled out with ripe, warm fruits and the sweet scents of country gardens and hedgerows, with gentle notes of musk and sandalwood. The blue-green, asymmetric glass bottle, smoothly-contoured like a water-polished pebble, was designed by Annegret Beier.

NOA

Launch: 1999
- ▲ Top note: White peony
- ▲ Middle notes: Blackcurrant leaves, Coffee
- ▲ Base notes: Musk, Benzoin, Frankincense

Style: A rounded fragrance of great depth and distinction, this has a luminous transparent quality, combining the pervasive milky fragrance of white peonies with the verdant freshness of blackcurrant leaves and a new, bitter-sweet coffee note never before used in perfumery, all underpinned with the intoxicating sensuality of musk. The bottle, designed by Beier, is a futuristic, clear crystal sphere, packaged in an ivory-coloured box that unfolds ingeniously like a flower opening its petals.

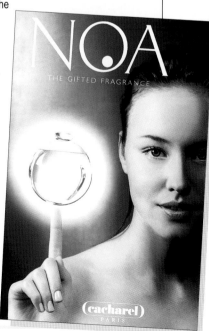

Right: The ad for Noa *maintains Cacharel's youthful image, but adds a touch of modern mystery and magic.*

FLORIS

Floris, the second-oldest perfumery in the world, has operated from the same premises in London for over 250 years, making bespoke perfumes as well as fragrances for the general public.

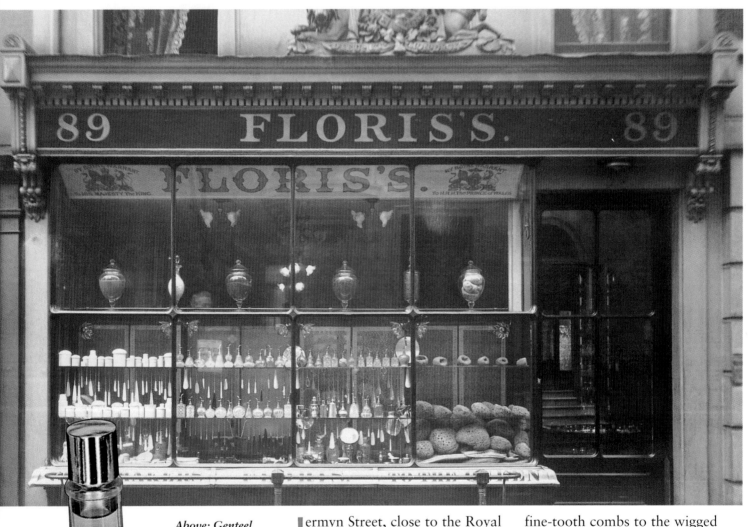

Above: Genteel traditions continue at the Jermyn St shop: customers are, for example, still handed their change on velvet change pads.
Left: No 89 for Men is a favourite of the Prince of Wales, who granted the store one of its two current Royal Warrants.

Jermyn Street, close to the Royal Court at St James's Palace and gentlemen's clubland in Pall Mall, was at the heart of fashionable 18th-century London. At No 89, almost opposite Wren's St James's Church, a young Menorcan called Juan Famenias Floris set up as a barber and comb-maker in 1730. He supplied ivory-handled shaving brushes, silver hatpins, toothbrushes, razor-straps and fine-tooth combs to the wigged and powdered dandies of the city.

FRAGRANCE PIONEER
The hardworking and thrifty Floris soon branched into perfumery, blending the essences and flower waters of his native Mediterranean into customized fragrances for his exclusive clientele. At that time, commercial perfumeries were a comparative novelty. As washing

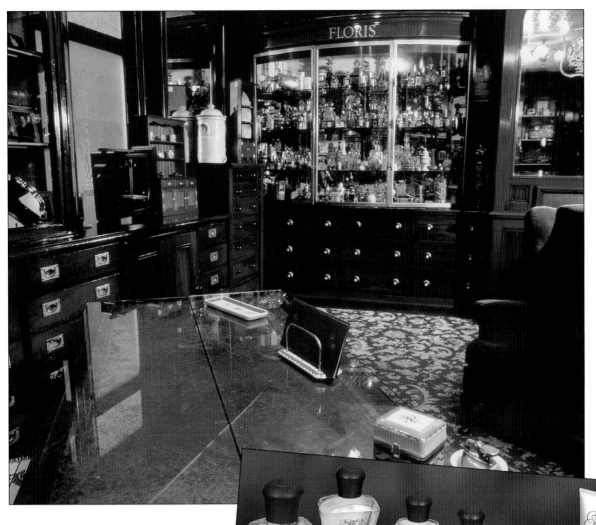

Below: As well as perfume and toilet waters, Floris make shaving and bath toiletries, pot-pourris and perfumed candles in their key fragrances.

was thought unhealthy, scents were used liberally in rooms and on clothes, gloves and fans to mask the resulting odours. Most scents were, in fact, made at home in domestic stillrooms to traditional recipes.

SCENTED COURT

It was the court of Louis XV in mid 18th-century France that made a cult of perfume, and the trend spread to England. The son of George III, later the Prince Regent, and Beau Brummell, the celebrated dandy, included a taste for perfume among their fashionable excesses; Brummell spent hours at Floris discussing the minutiae of his purchases. Where the Court shopped the gentry followed, and Floris's perfumery flourished. By 1800, well over 100 fragrances were being made in the shop's back room.

The patronage of the Prince began an association with the monarchy that continues to this day. When the Prince became George IV in 1820, he granted Floris its first Royal Warrant. It is now on display, with 16 others – the coveted warrants are reviewed every six years – at the Jermyn Street shop. Floris currently holds two, from the Queen and Prince Charles (said to be particularly fond of *No 89 for Men*).

Until the late 1960s, Floris fragrances were hand-crafted in the shop's basement, then packaged and sent upstairs to the shelves. At

109

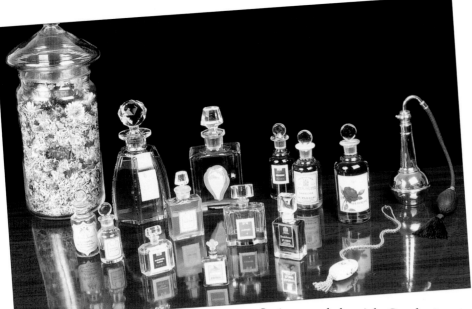

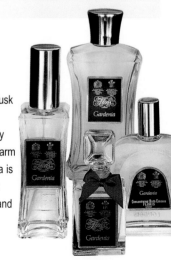

Right: Edwardian Bouquet, issued to celebrate Edward VII's accession in 1901, is still popular nearly 100 years later. *Left:* The Floris range is not advertised, but sells entirely on its reputation.

one time, many were tailored to a client's particular requirements, with the unique formulae recorded in the 'Specials' ledger. *Special No 127*, for example, now on general sale, was formulated for a Russian Grand Duke in 1890.

Fragrances first sold over 200 years ago are still available today, updated to modern tastes. Many of the scents are 'single-note' fragrances, formulated to enhance a dominant flower note, as in *Wild Hyacinth*, *Moss Rose* and *Limes*, launched in the late 19th century to combat the summer heat of the overcrowded city.

As well as the old favourites, Floris continues to produce new fragrances in the same tradition of excellence. The flowery *Florissa*, floral-oriental *Bouvardia*, lighter, green

Seringa and the rich *Gardenia* are among the most popular of the current female fragrances.

The London shop is still at 89 Jermyn Street, the oldest perfumery still in existence after Santa Maria Novella in Florence, and continues to be run by direct descendants of Juan Floris and his English wife Elizabeth Hodgkiss.

Floris

COLLECTION

FLORISSA

Launch: 1978
▲ Top notes: Lilac, Orange oil
▲ Middle notes: Rose, Jasmin, Lily-of-the-valley, Orris
▲ Base notes: Clove, Amber, Sandalwood

Style: This traditional floral fragrance is introduced by the fresh, captivating scent of lilac and sweet orange and combines the two classic notes of English rose and jasmin at the heart, swathed in the warm intensity of lily-of-the-valley and powdery orris root on a base of woody, ambery elements. It is very soft and feminine in a subtle, well-mannered, English sort of way, like flowing, flower-sprigged frocks with shady hats and snow-white lace gloves.

GARDENIA

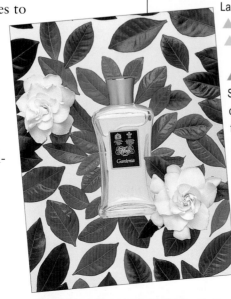

Launch: 1996
▲ Top notes: Bergamot, Neroli, Peach
▲ Middle notes: Gardenia, Ylang-ylang, Jasmin, Tuberose, Lily, Orange blossom, Cyclamen
▲ Base notes: Sandalwood, Labdanum, Balsam, Musk

Style: Inspired by an entry in one of Floris s 19th-century catalogues, *Gardenia* combines an intensely fragrant floral bouquet with fruity top notes and a warm sandal and resin base. The rich warmth of gardenia is softened by more delicate flowers so that it is light enough for day wear, yet it also has the richness and complexity to suit more glamorous occasions. Evocative of lazy summer days and warm starry nights, it is soft, enveloping, fresh and feminine.

Floris

PROFILE

1730 Juan Famenias Floris (right) opens a barber shop in Jermyn St, London.
1776 Juan hands over the business to his son.
1820 First Royal Warrant granted to Floris by George IV.
1851 Floris acquires its famous mahogany showcases from the Great Exhibition.
1862 Produces its first public catalogue of products.
1912 Regular shipments of Floris products to the USA begin.
1986 Floris shop opens in Madison Avenue, New York.
1995 Prince Charles commissions Floris to create the Highgrove Collection.
1999 Launches *At Home* collection of room scents, scented candles and other home fragrances.
2000 Floris products become available on the Internet.

PERFUME CHRONOLOGY

1700s *Lavender*	**1800s** *Limes*	**1890** *Special 127*	**1955** *No 89 for Men*	**1990** *Zinnia*
1700s *Lily of the Valley*	**1800s** *Moss Rose* (relaunched 1981)	**1901** *Edwardian Bouquet*	**1978** *Florissa*	**1992** *JF, Seringa*
1700s *Stephanotis*		(relaunched 1984)	**1979** *Elite*	**1994** *Bouvardia*
1700s *Rose Geranium*	**1835** *Wild Hyacinth*			**1996** *Gardenia*

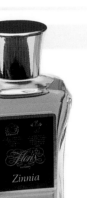

ZINNIA

Launch: 1990
△ Top notes: Violet, Galbanum, Ylang-ylang
△ Middle notes: Rose, Lily, Orris, Clove
△ Base notes: Sandalwood, Vanilla, Musk
Style: This oriental-style fragrance with the gentle pink colour of rosé wine was created by Floris's in-house perfumer, Douglas Cope, from an 1860 recipe in the Floris archive. Violet and ylang-ylang give an initial sweetness that dips into an intoxicating bouquet of summer flowers, with exotic spicy base notes — dominated by musk — giving a touch of excitement to the brew.

SERINGA

Launch: 1992
△ Top notes: Bergamot, Petitgrain, Mandarin, Mock orange blossom
△ Middle notes: Rose, Lilac, Lily-of-the-valley, Orchid, Ylang-ylang, Cyclamen
△ Base notes: Jasmin, Tuberose, Violet, Amber, Oakmoss, Musk
Style: This is a crisp, green-floral, vaguely oriental fragrance specifically designed by Douglas Cope to appeal to younger women with a more sophisticated, modern outlook. The lightly sharp, citrus top notes are fresh and exhilarating, paving the way for the much richer, headier floral heart, composed of English garden flowers and the more exotic blooms of orchid and ylang-ylang, and finishing with the sensuous touch of oriental tuberose, jasmin and musk.

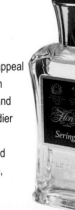

ight: Zinnia and Seringa, ke other fragrances in the Floris range, are sold in flaçons and s perfume sprays. Although Floris does not advertise, they do produce a colour catalogue of their products, which are now made in a factory in Devon. There are Floris shops in New York and Kobe, Japan, and the fragrances are exported worldwide.

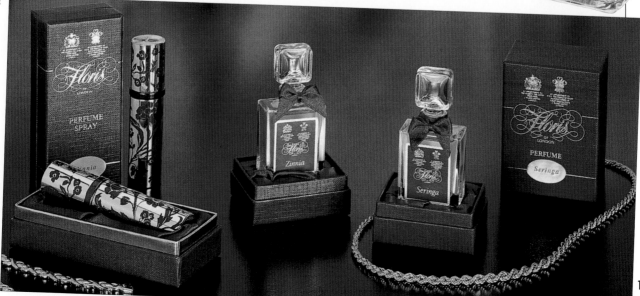

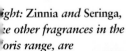

LANVIN

Lanvin is France's oldest established couture house, although it now concentrates on ready-to-wear. Its small range of fragrances includes one, Arpège, that is an acknowledged classic.

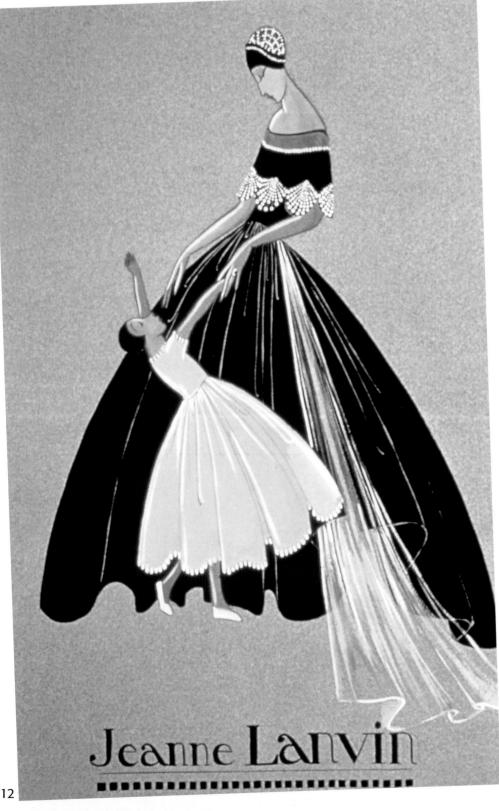

Jeanne Lanvin

The abiding passion and creative inspiration of Jeanne Lanvin's life was her daughter. Without Marie-Blanche, Jeanne's only child, there would have been no Lanvin, and no *Arpège*, one of the world's great perfumes. Marie-Blanche was an exquisite child, pretty, intelligent, charming and musically gifted. She inspired Jeanne's greatest creations and represented an ideal of carefree youth that Jeanne, the eldest of ten children, had never enjoyed.

She had worked from an early age, with a seamstress then a milliner. Jeanne was ambitious, hardworking and prodigiously talented. By the age of 18, with just one client, modest credit and her own boundless energy, she had

Left: The Lanvin logo by Paul Iribe expressed the mother and daughter bond at the heart of Lanvin. Right: Mon Péché (My Sin) was the first commercial Lanvin perfume.

MON PÉCHÉ
"MYSIN"
EXTRAIT DE
LANVIN
PARIS.   FRANCE

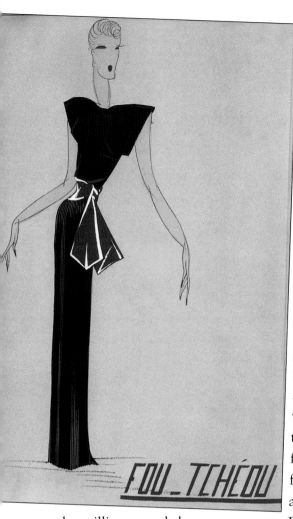

FOU_TCHÉOU

Left: In the 1930s, Jeanne designed elegant shifts with floating ribbons and stylized Art Deco appliqué, along with embroidered cocktail dresses.

daughters. In 1908 she opened a department especially for children's clothes, and a year later she was also dressing their mothers, specializing in matching mother-and-daughter outfits.

From the beginning, Jeanne stressed femininity and youthfulness, at any age. Although she herself mostly wore black with occasional touches of white, she favoured fantasy and romance.

Before World War I, she was famous for high-waisted Empire-style dresses with gilded embroidery and fabulous jewelled headdresses.

In 1918 Jeanne employed 800 people, and her premises included workrooms for tailored and semi-tailored clothes, lingerie, hats and embroidery, as well as a design studio. In 1920 she opened a new shop, taking over the whole of 15 rue du Faubourg-Saint-Honoré, the building where she had first been employed as a humble millinery assistant.

The shop was decorated in lavish style, with a gilded filigree lift cage, carved oak panels and spectacular bronze reliefs. The young designer Armand-Albert Rateau, who also decorated the interiors of her Paris mansion and villas at Cannes and Le Touquet, became a close friend of Jeanne. They completed various projects together, and it was Rateau who designed the famous spherical bottles used for all Lanvin perfumes, and particularly *Arpège*.

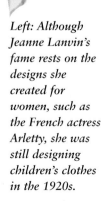

opened a millinery workshop. Four years later, in 1889, she had her own shop and a healthy list of well-heeled, fashionable clients.

SHORT MARRIAGE

Surprisingly perhaps, given her serious disposition, she married a dashing womanizer and gambler, Emilio de Pietro, who seduced her, it is said, for a bet. The marriage did not last, but it produced Marie-Blanche.

At that time, children wore scaled-down versions of adult clothes, but the dresses Jeanne made for Marie-Blanche – light, loose shapes, prettily embroidered and trimmed – entranced her millinery clients, who wanted similar garments for their own

Left: Although Jeanne Lanvin's fame rests on the designs she created for women, such as the French actress Arletty, she was still designing children's clothes in the 1920s.

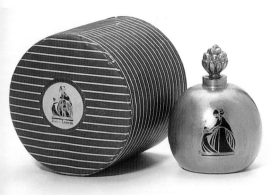

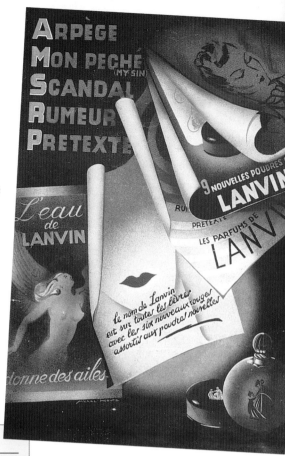

Right: In the 1930s, the Lanvin fragrance range was wider than now, but Arpége, *seen here in a gold bottle (left), has always been the star.*

Madame Zed, an elderly Russian perfumer, had already produced several exotically named, in-house fragrances for Lanvin couture clients, as well as *My Sin*, the company's first commercial scent,

which was a huge success in the USA. The commission for *Arpège* went to her successors, André Fraysse and Paul Vacher. Fraysse created a string of spectacular scents for Lanvin, such as *Scandale*, *Rumeur* and *Prétexte*. Only *Arpège* remains.

It had to be extra special. It was a 30th birthday present for Marie-Blanche, now the

Lanvin

1867	Jeanne Lanvin (below) born in Paris on 1 January.
1885	Opens her own milliner's workshop.
1895	Marries Emilio de Pietro.
1897	Daughter Marguerite (later Marie-Blanche) is born.
1903	Jeanne and Emilio are divorced.
1907	Marries journalist and diplomat Xavier Melet.
1908	Opens children's clothes department.
1909	Opens couture house.
1920	Meets interior designer Armand-Albert Rateau
1925	Marguerite marries Comte de Polignac; changes name to Marie-Blanche.
1925	First commercial perfume *My Sin* created by Madame Zed.
1946	Jeanne dies; Marie-Blanche takes over the running of Lanvin.
1958	Marie-Blanche dies.
1985	Maryll Lanvin, wife of Jeanne's great-nephew, takes over couture house.
1990	Lanvin acquired by L'Oréal.
1993	Lanvin gives up couture and concentrates on ready-to-wear.
1995	Ocimar Versolato becomes chief designer.
1998	Christina Ortiz, formerly of Prada, becomes chief designer.
1998	Flagship boutiques in Paris designed by Terence Conran.

P R O F I L E

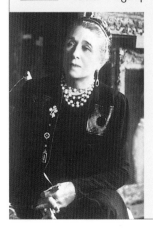

PERFUME CHRONOLOGY

1925 *Mon Péché/My Sin* (flaçon by Baccarat)	**1934** *Rumeur*
	1937 *Prétexte*
1927 *Arpège*	**1960** *Crescendo*
1928 *L'Ame Perdue/Lost Soul*	**1964** *Monsieur Lanvin*
	1964 *Vetyver*
1928 *Pétales Froissés*	**1981** *Lanvin for Men*
1931 *Scandale*	**1983** *Clair du Jour*
1933 *Eau de Lanvin*	**1998** *Lanvin L'Homme*

Comtesse de Polignac. Jeanne demanded 'a unique and timeless masterpiece'. Bernard Lanvin, her great-nephew, said she envisaged 'a magnificent perfume bouquet of pure natural flowers'.

CLASSIC CREATION

It took two years to develop. No expense was spared, and only the finest natural ingredients were used. It was named by Marie-Blanche, who felt it suggested an 'arpeggio', a cascade of musical notes. The glossy, spherical black bottle, with its gold raspberry stopper, carried the gilded Lanvin logo, created by artist Paul Iribe. This design, still used today, is a stylized Art Deco image of a mother and young daughter dressed for a ball, gazing into each other's eyes, with outstretched arms and clasped hands – a perfect loving symbol for a gift of love.

Lanvin
COLLECTION

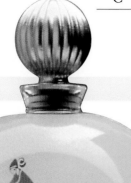

ARPÈGE

Launch: 1927

▲ Top notes: Aldehydes, Bergamot, Neroli, Coriander, Clove, Peach

▲ Middle notes: Orris, Jasmin, Rose, Ylang-ylang, Camellia, Lily-of-the-valley

▲ Base notes: Ambrein, Benzoin, Musk, Sandalwood, Patchouli, Vanilla, Vetiver

Style: This classic aldehydic, floral fragrance is ranked among the greatest perfumes of all time. André Fraysse's original formula contained over 60 natural essences, including rose, jasmin, delicate aromatic spices and potent animal elements, such as civet. The scent was reformulated and relaunched in 1993 and is currently Lanvin's only female fragrance. The perfume still uses many of the original ingredients, updated for modern tastes, but retains the spirit of the great classic, and is happily reunited with the glorious Art Deco flaçon designed by the artist Armand-Albert Rateau.

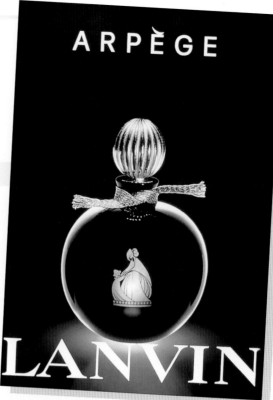

Above: Arpège is now marketed as a classic. This ad's background uses 'Lanvin blue', a colour specially created by Jeanne Lanvin.

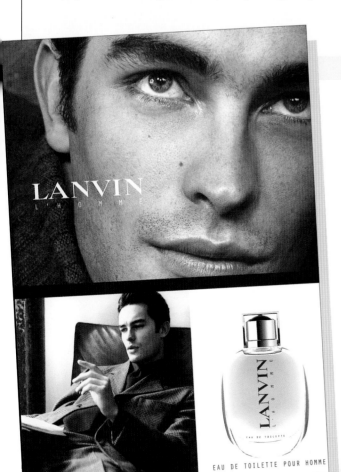

LANVIN L'HOMME

Launch: 1998

▲ Top notes: Citrus, Bergamot, Mandarin, Neroli

▲ Middle notes: Mint, Sage, Lavender, Pepper, Cardamom

▲ Base notes: Sandalwood, Musk

Style: Created by perfumer Alberto Morillas, this unashamedly masculine fragrance is contained in an elegant, clear glass 'hipflask' bottle with chrome flip-top cap, and packaged in 'Lanvin blue'. It is impeccably elegant and contemporary, with a distinct dash of the luxurious simplicity and easy confidence associated with superb natural materials. Its fresh, sharp citrus note is mellowed by enticing aromas of herbs and spices and anchored in the warm, woody appeal of sandalwood and musk. It evokes white cotton shirts, tactile raw linen and softest cashmere — absolutely pure, clean and natural, simply perfect but deeply sensual.

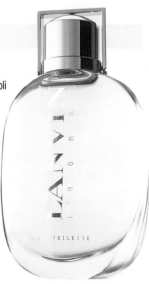

Left: Lanvin L'Homme is very much targeted at the young, modern, stylish man-about-town, as the advertising suggests.

MOSCHINO

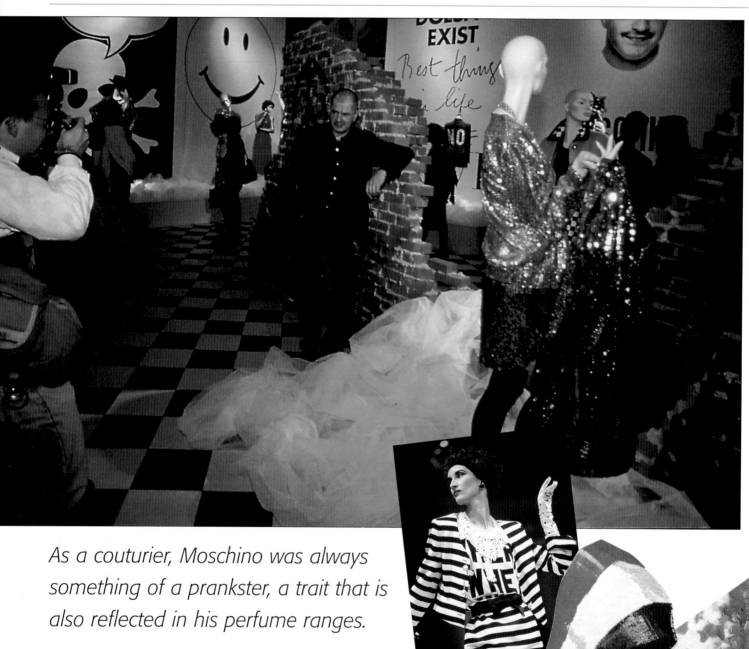

As a couturier, Moschino was always something of a prankster, a trait that is also reflected in his perfume ranges.

When he was 17, Franco Moschino ran away from his family home in a small town near Milan rather than join his father's iron foundry. He found work as a handyman. It was an inauspicious start to a dazzling and paradoxical career. By the time of his tragically early death in 1994, he had created one of the world's top-selling brands, with

Above: Moschino poses for the camera in an extravagant room setting designed for one of his shows. Right: Everything about Moschino – his clothes, logos, packaging and so on – shared the same essentially playful nature.

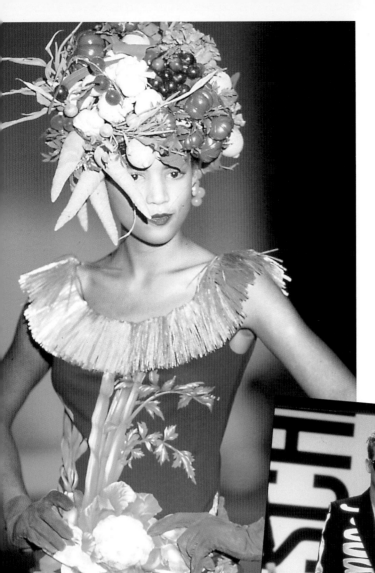

Left and below: Some of the garments in Moschino's couture style are extraordinarily camp, such as the Carmen Miranda-inspired dress on the left from his 1988 collection. The tradition has continued after his death; the skeleton suit below was part of the 1997–1998 autumn and winter collection.

Moschino was unpredictable, exciting and often brilliantly funny and surrealistic. He had an anarchic sense of humour and his shows were fabulous 'events', like a circus or carnival. At one of them, his models walked down the catwalk *en masse* dressed in huge Moschino carrier bags; at another they crawled like cats.

JOKER IN THE PACK

Moschino showed tops made entirely of safety pins, covered with condom packets, or with built-in coat-hangers or life-jackets; there was an 'organic' bikini seeded with grass that was allowed to grow; and a suit with the tailor's tacking still in place. Hats might be made of light bulbs, newspaper or wicker baskets, and jewellery of croissants, Q-Tips or furry teddy bears. Ballgowns were created from bin bags.

He loved to make fun of fashion clichés, such as the Chanel suit or Louis Vuitton suitcase (both companies sued), and also enjoyed witty slogans, such as 'Good Taste Doesn't Exist'; he adorned his clothes with English puns, such as 'Fashion Is Full of Chic', 'Waist of Money', 'Bull Chic' (on a matador jacket) and 'Ready to Where?' A straitjacket-style shirt was labelled 'For Fashion Victims Only'.

sales of over $200 million and nearly 4000 outlets worldwide.

In many ways, though, Moschino despised fashion. He took neither it nor himself seriously, and seized every opportunity to debunk its treasured icons, insult its most revered gurus and ridicule its most sacred illusions. At one show, he put moo-boxes on the gilt chairs of the world's most powerful fashion editors to mock their herd-like instincts, but the ruder and more provocative he was, the more people adored him.

Right: The distinctive flaçon designed for **Moschino pour Homme** *is a whisky bottle with two ends, presumably as a way of making it seem doubly masculine.*

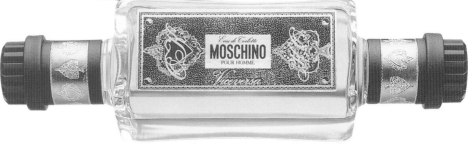

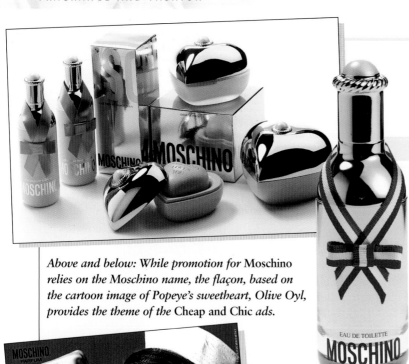

Above and below: While promotion for Moschino relies on the Moschino name, the flaçon, based on the cartoon image of Popeye's sweetheart, Olive Oyl, provides the theme of the Cheap and Chic ads.

Moschino
COLLECTION

MOSCHINO

Launch: 1987

▲ Top notes: Galbanum, Tagetes, Freesia, Honeysuckle, Plum

▲ Middle notes: Gardenia, Rose, Ylang-ylang, Clove, Nutmeg, Pepper, Sandalwood, Patchouli

▲ Base notes: Musk, Amber, Vanilla

Style: This classic floral-oriental fragrance has rich, fruity, aromatic top notes and a flowery, spicy heart. The overall effect is sexy, provocative and lightly exotic, evoking sophistication and up-to-the-minute style with a dash of rebelliousness. The bottle, designed by Pierre Dinand, resembles a wine bottle draped with the Italian tricolour ribbon, and has a silvery chrome cap with an earring-like pearl on top. The launch ads featured a model apparently drinking the scent from the bottle through a straw.

CHEAP AND CHIC

Launch: 1996

▲ Top notes: Bergamot, Petitgrain, Yuzu lemon, Rosewood

▲ Middle notes: Water-lily, Cyclamen, Rose, Jasmin, Peony, Violet

▲ Base notes: Orris, Sandal, Vetiver, Vanilla, Tonka bean, White orchid, Amber

Style: Designed to go with Moschino's youthful Cheap and Chic collections, this fragrance bursts with freshness and vitality. Lemony top notes are filled out and given depth with richly scented, sensuous floral elements and a woody-musky base, with a vaporous spiral of white orchid and vanilla to finish. Some of the ingredients were obtained by headspace technology. The 'Olive Oyl' bottle devised by the Moschino team is a typical visual joke.

There was also a serious side to Moschino. As well as the styles designed to shock, he created a steady stream of sexy clothes that were flattering, fun to wear and always immaculately made. He was never an élitist, and was one of the first designers to introduce an affordable range, Cheap and Chic, in 1988. Moschino supported animal rights and environmentalist causes: his Fur for Fun fake fur collection in 1988 signalled his views on the fur trade,

and in 1994 he showed his first Ecouture collection and introduced a 'Nature-Friendly Garment' label. The Franco Moschino Foundation, set up after his death, continues to provide help for HIV-positive children in Italy and Romania.

FRAGRANCE WITH A SMILE
Moschino fragrances reflect his zany, irreverent humour. *Moschino*, a classic floral-oriental perfume, was launched in 1987, followed by

Right: As well as their outrageous sense of fun, Moschino clothes are also renowned for their colour and dash.

Moschino pour Homme, packaged in a double-ended 'whisky' bottle, and *Cheap and Chic*, a sparkling fruity-flowery scent, as youthful and informal as the clothes.

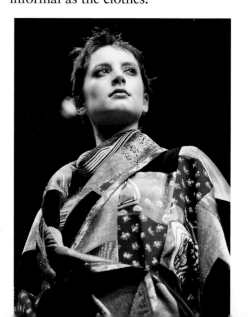

OH! DE MOSCHINO

Launch: 1996

▲ Top notes: Citrus notes, Tangerine, Bergamot, Rosewood

▲ Middle notes: Lotus, Cyclamen, Yellow flag iris, Water-lily, Peony, Lily-of-the-valley, Stephanotis

▲ Base notes: Heliotrope, Hawthorn, Orris, Sandalwood, Musk

Style: An eau de toilette with staying power, *Oh! de Moschino* is fresh, young and light, but with enough body for wearing all year round. Clear, sharp, citrus top notes give way to the shimmering scents of aquatic blossoms – lotus, lily and yellow flag – and blend intriguingly into the headier sensuality of heliotrope, orris and musk. The flaçon is the same wine bottle shape as the original *Moschino,* but the glass is frosted and draped with a blue ribbon 'sealed' with a red heart.

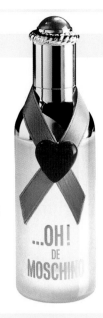

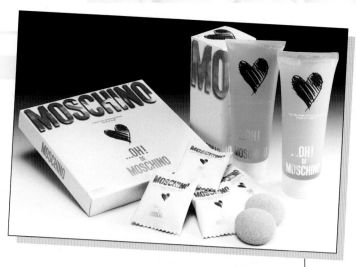

Above and below: Oh! de Moschino *and* Uomo?, *like other Moschino fragrances, are available in a wide range of scented toiletries.*

UOMO?

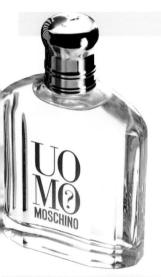

Launch: 1999

▲ Top notes: Hedione, Rosewood, Coriander, Kumquat

▲ Middle notes: Cyclamen, Cinnamon, Clary sage

▲ Base notes: Cedarwood, Artemisia, Amber wood, Musk

Style: This zesty, fresh, spicy, aromatic-floral fragrance combines virility with a generous, warm heart, and expresses overtly the sexual ambiguity that accompanies the idea of the 1990s' 'new man'. The classy, clear glass bottle is in the shape of a hip flask with a silver screw top, a traditional emblem of masculinity; the question mark inside the final 'O' of Uomo introduces the doubt.

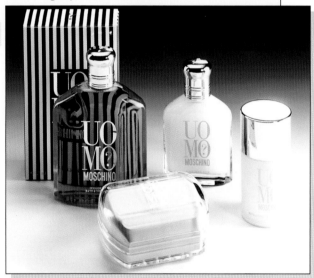

Oh! de Moschino is a lighter, *eau fraîche* variation of the original *Moschino*, packaged in the same wine bottle shape but draped, this time, with a bright red heart instead of an Italian flag.

Uomo? (Man?), the most recent men's fragrance, exemplifies, with its eloquent question mark, the ambiguity wafting through the whole idea of virility in male perfumes. It is yet another example of the distinctive Moschino knack of highlighting serious issues through the medium of apparently frivolous pranks.

PROFILE

Moschino

1950 Franco Moschino (below) born in Abbiategrasso, Milan province, Italy.

1972-77 Works as an illustrator for Versace.

1983 Founds own company, Moonshadow; launches Moschino label with first womenswear collection.

1986 Introduces first menswear collection in Milan.

1987 Launches first perfume *Moschino*.

1990 Launches the 'Stop the Fashion System' ad campaign.

1991 Launches Moschino Parfums in New York.

1994 18 September, Moschino dies of heart attack; company continues under direction of Rossella Jardini.

1995 Franco Moschino Foundation set up to help HIV-positive children in Italy and Romania.

PERFUME CHRONOLOGY

1987	*Moschino*	**1996**	*Oh! de*
1989	*Moschino for Men*		*Moschino*
1996	*Cheap and Chic*	**1999**	*Uomo?*

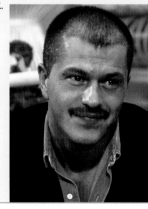

AVON

Avon's direct-selling methods, employing women world-wide, have made it one of the largest international cosmetic houses. It is a woman-centred business, with 86 per cent of its executives and virtually all its representatives female.

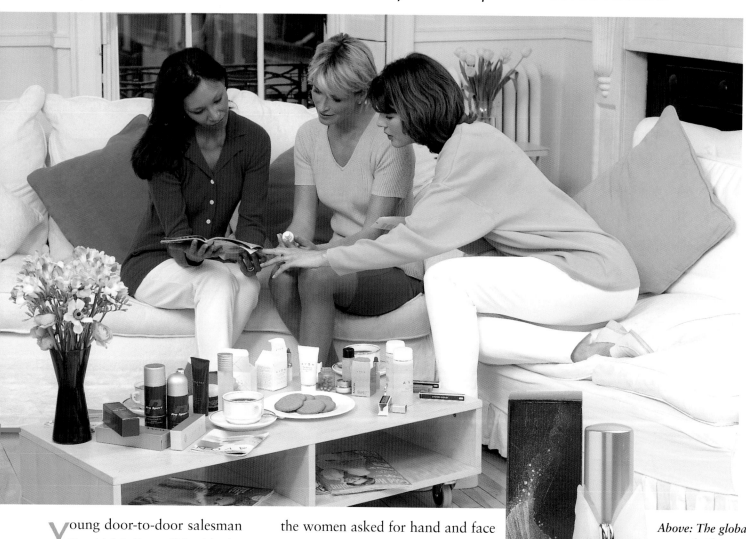

Above: The global network of some 2.8 million Avon ladies selling its products makes the company unique. Left: Evermore (1989) is a fragrance combining rose, ylang-ylang, musk, sandal and amber.

Young door-to-door salesman David McConnell had little luck hawking bibles around rural New York State in the 1880s. The farmers' wives were unimpressed. One eventually told him: 'If only you would bring us real perfume from Paris, then we would buy.'

McConnell took the hint, and came back a few weeks later with 'Paris perfume' – made in California. Sales were good, and the women asked for hand and face creams, scented soaps and talcum powder – in fact, everything their husbands inevitably forgot to buy on their trips to town.

A NEW MISSION
McConnell abandoned the bible business, commissioned chemists to devise some formulas, leased an aircraft hangar as a factory and hired two workers. The California

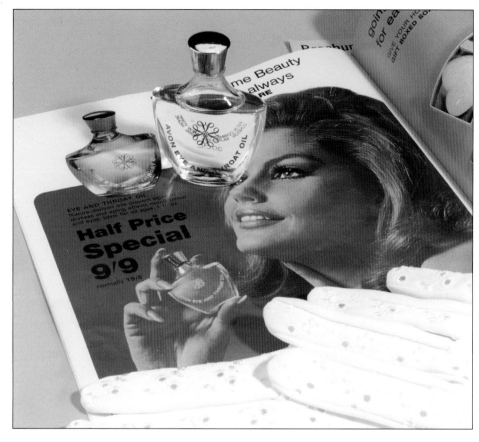

Above: Avon's catalogues are its sole selling tool. This one is from the early 1960s, when the company had just started up in Britain, where there are now 160,000 Avon ladies.
Below right: Avon regularly updates its cosmetics ranges in line with fashion.

Perfume Company was born. Years later, after a trip to Stratford-upon-Avon, he changed the company name to Avon, a word that he felt could easily be pronounced in many languages; by that time, his ambitions had become global. Today, Avon is the world's leading direct-seller of cosmetics and beauty products, with close to $5 billion of sales each year in a total of 135 countries.

Its enormous success owes much to its unique selling system. It was pioneered by Mrs P Albee of Winchester, New Hampshire, one of McConnell's original housewife customers and effectively the first 'Avon lady'.

Avon products were, and still are, sold by female sales reps who visit customers in their homes,

strictly by appointment and with cast-iron, money-back guarantees. They show the products and explain how to use them, take orders and deliver the goods personally – which provides another chance to show new products and take new orders. And so the process continues.

A SPECIAL RELATIONSHIP

The particular effectiveness of Avon ladies stems from the relationships they build up with their customers, gaining their confidence and providing welcome friendly contact for women who might be isolated in their homes, whether on rural farmsteads or urban housing estates.

They are housewives selling to housewives in the cosy, familiar surroundings of their own living rooms. Potentially intimidating encounters with glamorous – and sometimes brittle – salesgirls on department store cosmetics counters can be avoided.

As well as suiting the customers, the system has advantages for the

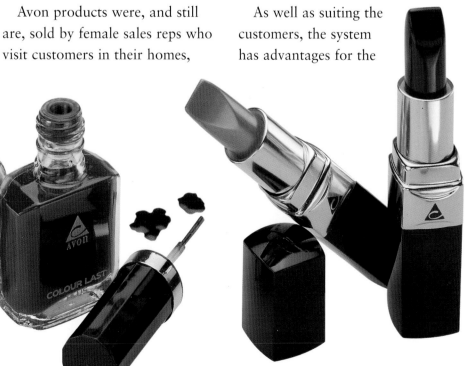

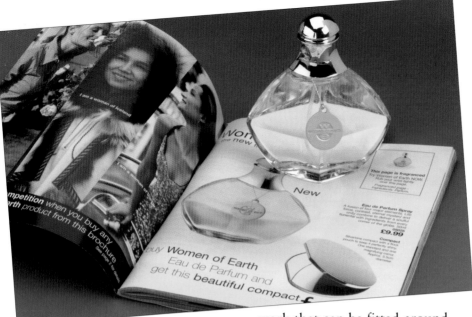

Left: Today, Avon catalogues have over 100 pages and include a wide range of products, as well as cosmetics and perfumes.

they are nevertheless quality products that make use of the latest research and technology.

RADICAL INNOVATIONS

In products such as Perfecting Face Complex and Anew, they pioneered the inclusion of AHA (alpha hydroxy acid) and vitamins A and C in skin care. The latest perfume *Perceive* (1999) uses up-to-date, mood-enhancing aromachological techniques, and includes synthesised pheromones.

Avon ladies. In the early days, when women were not expected to work outside the home, it gave them financial independence. Even today, it provides

work that can be fitted around home and family.

Over the past 110 years or so, thousands of items have passed through the pages of the Avon catalogue, the Avon lady's 'bible'. Although not the glitziest of goods,

Avon products now include gifts, toys, costume jewellery, lingerie, porcelain, glassware, CDs

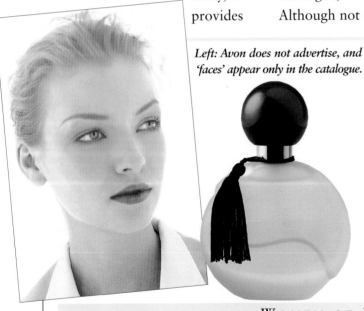

Left: Avon does not advertise, and 'faces' appear only in the catalogue.

Avon
C O L L E C T I O N

FAR AWAY

Launch: 1995

▲ Top notes: Jasmin, Freesia, Ylang-ylang
▲ Middle notes: Osmanthus, Orange blossom, Peach
▲ Base notes: Precious woods, Vanilla, Musk

Style: This scent expresses a gentle sophistication, suitable for everyday wearing, with an appealing bouquet of fragrant tropical flowers and rich fruity elements. It is packaged in a simple, elegant, round clear bottle topped with a bright pink stopper and draped with a silky tassel.

WOMEN OF EARTH

Launch: 1998

▲ Top notes: Kadota fig leaves, fruit and branch, Orange, Bergamot
▲ Middle notes: Apple blossom, Sweet pea, Winter daphne, Snowdrop, Jasmin
▲ Base notes: Vanilla, Amber, Peach, Musk, Sandalwood

Style: This fruity-floral fragrance combines the luscious juicy scents of ripe Mediterranean fruits with the soft perfume of spring and summer flowers. The green woody sweetness of figs tinged with cool citrus aromas from orange and bergamot blend into the gentle freshness of English snowdrops, sweet pea and apple blossom, and are given a lightly exotic, more sensuous edge with Chinese winter daphne and Egyptian jasmin. The spicy, fruity base adds a soft enveloping warmth, length and depth to the mixture.

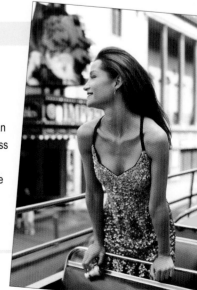

Avon

1886	Door-to-door bible salesman David McConnell (right) begins selling perfumes in the USA as The California Perfume Company.
1887	Mrs P Albee pioneers the company's unique direct-selling method.
1939	The company name is changed to Avon.
1959	Avon moves into the UK market.
1987	Avon's Women of Enterprise progamme is launched.
1989	Avon becomes the first major beauty company to stop using animals in safety testing.
1993	The Avon Breast Awareness Crusade and Avon Worldwide Fund for Women's Health are launched.
1997	Avon becomes the first major beauty company to sell its goods online through a global website.

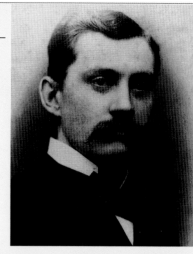

PERFUME CHRONOLOGY

1964	Occur!	**1982**	Odyssey	**1989**	Evermore	**1994**	Oliver Strelli	**1997**	Josie; Starring
1966	Elegance	**1982**	Black Suede	**1989**	Facets	**1995**	Rare Gold;	**1998**	Women of Earth
1968	Charisma	**1985**	Ophelia	**1992**	Perle Noire		Natori; Far Away	**1999**	Rare Rubies;
1971	Moonwind	**1986**	Fifth Avenue	**1993**	Reve Voilé	**1996**	Millennia		Perceive

and videos, as well as cosmetics, skin care toiletries and fragrances. Well made and affordable, they are some of the most widely used make-up and perfume items around. Surveys show that a staggering 90 per cent of American women have used Avon products at least once in their lifetime, while more beauty products carry the unassuming Avon brand name than any other in the world.

RARE RUBIES

Launch: 1999

▲ Top notes: Orange flower, Bergamot, Artemisia, Clementine, Freesia, Ylang-ylang, Coriander, Ginger, Pimento

▲ Middle notes: Cinnamon, Nutmeg, Carnation, Rose, Peony, Lily, Jasmin

▲ Base notes: Sandalwood, Amber, Musk, Cedarwood, Vanilla

Style: This spicy-oriental fragrance, based on the glamour and passion symbolized by rubies, the rarest of gems, combines rich floral ingredients with exotic spices. Citrus top notes blend with sensuous ylang-ylang flowers, while touches of hot ginger and pimento provide spiciness; in the heart are alluring floral scents and warm mellow notes, which merge into long-lasting vanilla and a woody, ambery base.

Women of ... promotes ...niversality ...mininity. ...: Rare ...es' image ...ises opulence ...excitement.

PERCEIVE

Launch: 1999

▲ Top notes: Freesia, White pepper, Gardenia

▲ Middle notes: Ylang-ylang, Damascus plum, Carnation, Pear

▲ Base notes: Vanilla, Musk, Cedarwood, Sandalwood

Style: The first Avon fragrance with specific mood-elevating ingredients was created by British perfumer Christopher Sheldrake to promote relaxation, confidence and focus. It fuses five harmonious accords with synthesised pheromones in a radiant oriental-style perfume composed of sparkling, look-alive top notes, a spicy, warm core of ripe fruits and exotic flowers, with more tranquil elements in the base. The multi-faceted bottle is inspired by natural quartz crystal, said to possess semi-mystical qualities linked to energy and harmony.

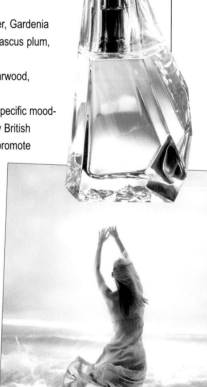

Right: Mystical, New-Age imagery emphasizes Perceive's mood-enhancing qualities.

CARON

Caron, founded in 1903 by a visionary amateur perfumer, is a Paris fragrance house that has issued many high-quality perfumes throughout the 20th century, including several classics.

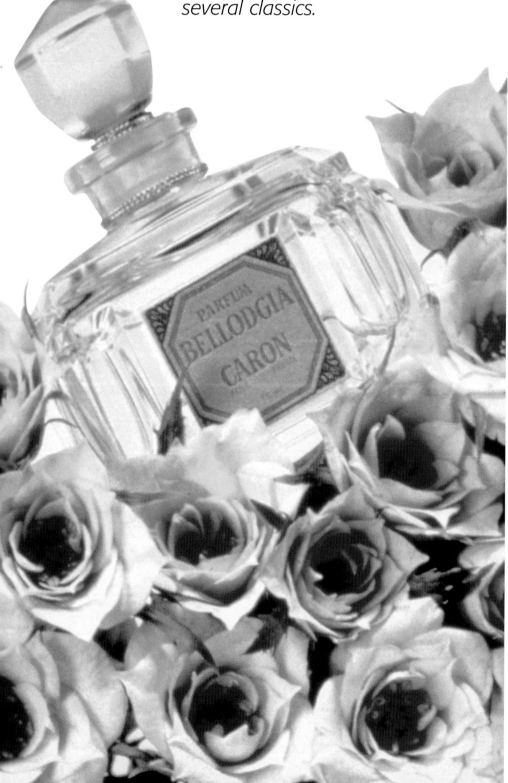

The original Caron perfume house was an unassuming boutique in the rue Rossini in Paris. In 1903 it caught the eye of Ernest Daltroff, a perfumer looking for a French-sounding label for his new products. He built Caron into one of the most successful perfumeries in France, producing more scents than any other prestige house. It is now one of the last of the great Parisian houses devoted entirely to fragrance.

Caron combined two remarkable talents – Daltroff, an instinctively brilliant 'nose', and Félicie Vanpouille, a dressmaker, who designed most of the flaçons and supervised the presentation of virtually every fragrance until her retirement in 1967, aged 94.

UNUSUAL RELATIONSHIP

The pair were lovers, but although she was referred to in the company as 'Madame', Vanpouille refused to marry Daltroff. When they separated, after more than 30 years, she married someone else.

Their professional ties were stronger, though. When growing anti-semitism forced Daltroff, a Jew, to leave France for Canada in 1939, he gave Vanpouille total control of the business.

Left: Ernest Daltroff created Bellodgia *(1927) to remind Félicie Vanpouille of the Italian town of Bellagia, which she loved. Rose, jasmin and violet lie at its heart. The flaçon is by Baccarat.*

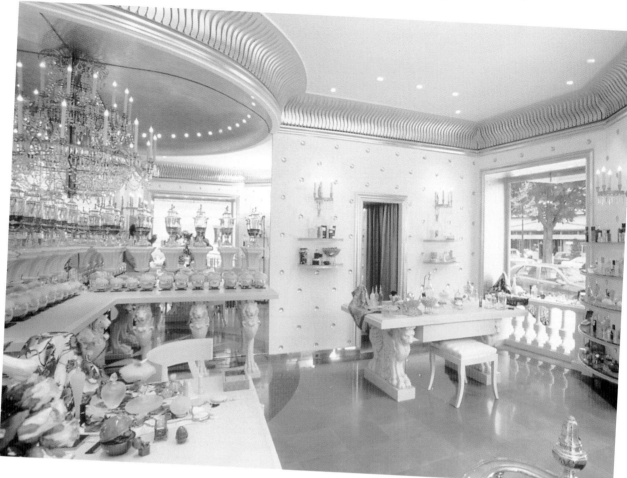

Right: In the Caron 'temple of perfume' in Paris's avenue Montaigne, perfumes are displayed like jewels on bevelled glass shelves, and gilt-framed mirrors reflect the huge Baccarat crystal urns from which the precious essences are decanted into gleaming bottles. Below: The single-note perfume Muguet de Bonheur (1952), based entirely around lily-of-the-valley, has a bright, youthful freshness.

Her sure sense of style and unorthodox imagination perfectly complemented his impetuous genius. He was bursting with fragrance ideas, inspired largely by childhood travels in the Middle East, Europe and the Americas. They had left him with a store of vivid memories, including the tantalizing piquancy of unfamiliar spices and the heady scent of exotic tropical flowers.

The re-creation of these scent memories in fragrances became his lifelong passion. Vanpouille helped to spark and channel his ideas, and devised evocative names, packages and images in perfect harmony with the changing spirit of the times.

FIRST SUCCESSES

Their first big success was *Narcisse Noir* (1911), a langorous, sensual fragrance based on rose, jasmin and orange blossom, and presented in a Baccarat crystal bottle. It was immortalized by the American actress Gloria Swanson in the film *Sunset Boulevard*; it was her favourite perfume in real life.

One of the most original creations, *Tabac Blond* (1919), was inspired by the type of tobacco used by Allied troops in World War I. It was dedicated to the flappers and their cigarette-smoking habits, although its leather and tobacco tones seemed more suited to men.

Next came *Nuit de Noël* (1922), the company's triumphant début in the USA. *En Avion* (1930) was a celebration of the exploits of the first female aviators. Vanpouille's elegant Art Deco flaçon helped glamorize the growing vogue for air travel. Another exquisite Art Deco piece held *Fleur de Rocaille*, Caron's best-selling perfume in the USA for many years.

When Daltroff fled the growing threat of the Nazis, he left Vanpouille in charge of business at Caron, with his assistant 'nose'

Right: Félicie Vanpouille was responsible with Daltroff for creating the Caron reputation. Far right: Infini *(1970) has a bottle by Serge Mansau.*

Michel Morsetti as chief perfumer. Daltroff died of cancer two years later in New York.

FRAGRANT LEGACY
Despite a stormy relationship with Vanpouille, now Mme Bergaud, Morsetti stayed for over 20 years. Daltroff had left him literally hundreds of

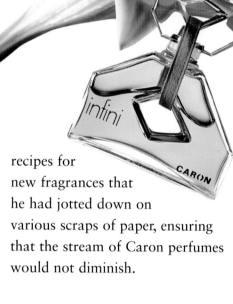

recipes for new fragrances that he had jotted down on various scraps of paper, ensuring that the stream of Caron perfumes would not diminish.

A MODERN COMPANY
Among the triumphs of this post-war torrent of new fragrances were *With Pleasure* (1949), Andy Warhol's choice; *Muguet de Bonheur* (1952), a youthful single-flower fragrance; *Montaigne* (1966), the last word in luxury and elegance; the consciously modern *Infini* (1970), with its sparkling green top notes and aldehydic heart; and *Nocturnes* (1981), which echoed in its dark sensuality the old black magic of *Nuit de Noël*.

In 1982, a new Caron temple of perfume opened in the prestigious avenue Montaigne in Paris. Stylish, sumptuous, yet discreet, it is a fitting memorial to Caron's magnificent past and an emblem of its gloriously self-confident present.

PROFILE

Caron

1903 Company founded by Ernest Daltroff.
1904 Daltroff (below left) creates first Caron perfume, *Radiant*.
1905 Daltroff moves to rue de la Paix and meets Félicie Vanpouille.
1922 Daltroff gives Vanpouille a half-share in the business.
1939 Daltroff leaves Vanpouille in charge of Caron.
1941 Daltroff dies in New York; 'nose' Michel Morsetti takes over as perfumer with Vanpouille still sole proprietor.
1962 Vanpouille (now Mme Bergaud) sells the company to Revillon but continues to be involved in Caron until her retirement.
1965 Morsetti retires.
1966 Mme Bergaud opens a luxurious boutique in the place Vendôme.
1967 Mme Bergaud retires at 94.
1970 The company is taken over by US pharmaceutical company Robins.
1982 A new Caron 'temple of perfume' opens in avenue Montaigne, Paris.

PERFUME CHRONOLOGY

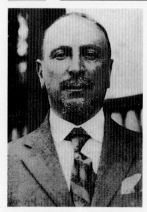

1904	*Radiant*	**1947**	*Farnesiana*
1909	*Chantecler*	**1949**	*Rose; Or et Noir; With Pleasure*
1911	*Narcisse Noir*		
1912	*L'Infini*	**1952**	*Muguet de Bonheur*
1916	*N'Aimez Que Moi*	**1954**	*Poivre*
1919	*Tabac Blond*	**1966**	*Montaigne*
1922	*Nuit de Noël*	**1970**	*Infini*
1924	*Acaciosa*	**1976**	*Yatagan*
1927	*Bellodgia; Le Pois de Senteur*	**1981**	*Nocturnes*
		1985	*Le No 3*
1930	*En Avion*	**1990**	*Parfum Sacré*
1933	*Fleur de Rocaille*	**1995**	*Eau de Cologne de Caron*
1934	*Pour un Homme*		
1941	*Royal Bain de Champagne*	**1996**	*Eau de Caron Pure*
		1997	*Aimez-Moi*

Caron

C O L L E C T I O N

NUIT DE NOËL

Launch: 1922

▲ Top notes: Jasmin, Ylang-ylang, Rose

▲ Middle notes: Violet leaves, Lily-of-the-valley, Orris, Tuberose

▲ Base notes: Sandalwood, Vetiver, Mousse de Saxe

Style: One of Daltroff's archetypal spicy-oriental fragrances, this subtle cocktail of exuberant aromatic notes is designed to evoke the warm, festive atmosphere of Christmas Eve, and is redolent of the scents of snug furs, leaping flames and smouldering incense. It is flowery, but also musky and earthy. The elegant black glass flaçon designed by Vanpouille carries a gold 'flapper' band. The atomizer is in an equally stylish bottle which picks up the flapper motif (above).

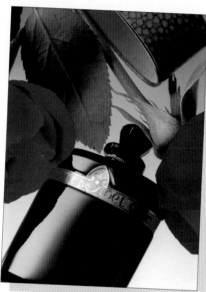

Above: The promotion for Nuit de Noël *highlights its rose scent.*

PARFUM SACRÉ

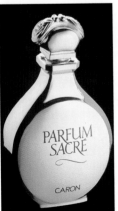

Launch: 1990

▲ Top notes: Pepper, Cinnamon, Lavender, Coriander

▲ Middle notes: Clove, Rose, Jasmin, Orange blossom

▲ Base notes: Mimosa, Myrrh, Musk, Amber, Vanilla

Style: The name, echoing the ancient, sacred origins of perfume as temple incense, is appropriate because *Parfum Sacré* has a mysterious, timeless, oriental quality, with a piercing, spicy intensity that heralds a deeply sensual heart, itself dominated by the intoxicating scents of jasmin and rose absolute. The overall effect is opulent, utterly confident and completely feminine.

Right: The advertising for Aimez-Moi *(Love Me) has the same self-confidence as its name – more command than plea.*

FLEUR DE ROCAILLE

Launch: 1933 (relaunched 1993)

▲ Top notes: Gardenia, Violet, Lilac, Aldehydes

▲ Middle notes: Rose, Jasmin, Orris, Mimosa, Lily-of-the-valley, Carnation, Ylang-ylang

▲ Base notes: Sandalwood, Cedar, Amber, Musk, Oakmoss

Style: A classic floral-fougère fragrance once described by couturier Karl Lagerfeld as 'the best perfume ever made', *Fleur de Rocaille* was inspired by Monet's paintings of water-lillies and has a similar close harmony of elements with no single dominant note. An opulent bouquet of natural flower scents enhanced by aldehydes, it is both fragile and potent, exuding youthful vivacity and a radiant underlying sensuality.

Right: Flowers and femininity are the key to advertising Fleur de Rocaille.

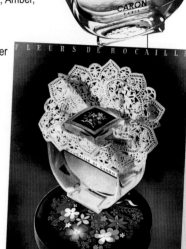

AIMEZ-MOI

Launch: 1997

▲ Top notes: Bergamot, Anise, Caraway, Cardamom, Violet leaf, Magnolia, Freesia, Mint

▲ Middle notes: Jasmin, Orris, Peach, Lily-of-the-valley, Rose, Osmanthus, Heliotrope, Tonka beans, Vanilla

▲ Base notes: Clove, Amber, Musk, Precious woods

Style: This resolutely modern, woody-floral fragrance has arrestingly spicy anise and bergamot top notes melting through a complex accord into a sumptuous floral bouquet tinged with a peachy lusciousness and the sweet warmth of vanilla. The finish is a classic lingering dry-down of amber and precious woods. Assertive and seductive, yet tender, it evokes the radiant self-confidence of those who are truly loved, and is a genuine original.

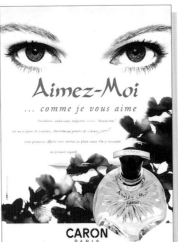

Picture Acknowledgments

Cover: Cecil Beaton/Camera Press, L. Parker/Orbis; 6 Courtesy Givenchy Parfums; 8l Camera Press, 8r courtesy Armani; 9 Farabolafoto, 9 (inset) courtesy Armani, 9r Camera Press; 10l Advertising Archives, 10r IGDA; 11r Advertising Archives, 11tl & c IGDA, 11bl Farabolafoto; 12t Cecil Beaton Archive, courtesy of Sotheby's, London, 12 (inset) Rex Features; 13l Sygma, 13r Camera Press; 14tl Sygma, 14tr Glöss Verlag, 14br Advertising Archives; 15tc Glöss Verlag, 15tr Advertising Archives, 15lc Roberto Fusconi, 15c courtesy Chanel, 15bl Glöss Verlag, 15br Advertising Archives; 16 courtesy Estée Lauder; 17l Advertising Archives, 17r courtesy Estée Lauder; 18t courtesy Estée Lauder, 18b Advertising Archives; 19tr & bl Advertising Archives, 19tl, cc, cr & br courtesy Estée Lauder; 20 courtesy Archives Christian Dior; 21t & tr Rex Features, 21b courtesy Christian Dior, 22bl & br Advertising Archives, 22tl, c & r courtesy Christian Dior; 23tl & bl Advertising Archives, 23r courtesy Christian Dior; 24bl courtesy Kenzo, 24tr Steve Wood/Rex Features; 25 tl and tr courtesy Kenzo, 25bl Barthelemy/Rex Features, 25br Charlotte Macpherson/Camera Press; 26tl and cr courtesy Kenzo/Kenneth Green Associates, 26bl and br Advertising Archives; 27tl and c courtesy Kenzo/ Kenneth Green Associates, 27tc and tr Vintage Magazine Company, 27bl courtesy Kenzo; 28bl Advertising Archives, 28tr Ben Coster/Camera Press, 29bl Sipa Press/Rex Features, 29tr Ben Coster/Camera Press; 30bl Sipa Press/Rex Features, 30 Advertising Archives, 30br courtesy Yves Saint-Laurent; 31all courtesy Yves Saint-Lauren; 32bl courtesy Calvin Klein Cosmetics, 32tr Charlotte Macpherson/Camera Press; 33tl courtesy Calvin Klein Cosmetics, 33bl Richard Open/Camera Press, 33r Charlotte Macpherson/Camera Press; 34all courtesy Calvin Klein Cosmetics; 35all courtesy Calvin Klein Cosmetics; 36 courtesy Benetton; 37 all courtesy Benetton; 38tl Sipa Press/Rex Features, 38tr & bl courtesy Benetton; 39tr & mr Advertising Archives, 39 rest courtesy Benetton; 40t Sipa Press/Rex Features, 40b courtesy Parfum Givenchy, 41t Ben Kosta/Camera Press, 41b Sipa Press/Rex Features; 42bl Advertising Archives, 42 remaining pics courtesy Parfum Givenchy; 43 all courtesy Parfum Givenchy; 44 all courtesy Lancôme; 45 all courtesy Lancôme; 46ml & bl Advertising Archives, 46 remaining pics courtesy Lancôme; 47mr Advertising Archives, 47 remaining pics courtesy Lancôme; 48 all courtesy Guerlain; 49t G. Neri/S. Benbow, 49mr courtesy Guerlain, 49b Farabolafoto; 50 all courtesy Guerlain; 51 all courtesy Guerlain; 52t Rex Features/Frederic Steven, 52b courtesy Kenneth Green Associates; 53t Rex Features/Helena Christensen, 53b Farabolafoto; 54tl & ml Advertising Archives, 54tm courtesy Jean Paul Gaultier Parfum, 54mr courtesy Kenneth Green Associates, 54b courtesy Jean Paul Gaultier; 55tl & b courtesy Kenneth Green Associates, 55tr Advertising Archives, 55ml courtesy Jean Paul Gaultier Parfum; 56 both courtesy Elizabeth Arden; 57 all courtesy Elizabeth Arden; 58 all courtesy Elizabeth Arden; 59tr Advertising Archives, 59tl, ml, mr, bl & br courtesy Elizabeth Arden; 60t & b courtesy Versace; 61tl Rex Features/Steve Wood; 62tr Rex Features-Sipa, 62ml Advertising Archives, 62ml & br courtesy Versace; 63tl, mr & bm courtesy Versace, 63ml & br Advertising Archives; 64t & r courtesy Jean Patou; 65 all courtesy Jean Patou; 66 all courtesy Jean Patou; 67tr & bl Advertising Archives, 67tl, ml, mr & br courtesy Jean Patou; 68t IGDA, 68m Rex Features/Sipa Press; 69t Topham PicturePoint, 69r Rex Features/Sipa Press; 70tm, mr & b IGDA, 70tl & ml Advertising Archives; 71tm & ml IGDA, 71tr Advertising Archives, 71mr courtesy Gucci, 71bl Rex Features/Tom Ford; 72l Rex Features/Steve Wood, 72r courtesy Kenneth Green Associates; 73r Rex Features/Steve Wood, 73bl courtesy Kenneth Green Associates; 74tl, tr & bl Kenneth Green Associates, 74br Advertising Archives; 75tl, tr & m courtesy Kenneth Green Associates, 75tr Advertising Archives; 76tl courtesy Nina Ricci, 76bl & br IGDA; 77tl courtesy Nina Ricci, 77m courtesy Nina Ricci/Joe Dorsey; 78m & br courtesy Nina Ricci, 78tr Creative Fragrances, 78ml courtesy Nina Ricci/Tony Kaye, 78bl Advertising Archives; 79tl & bm courtesy Nina Ricci, 79ml IGDA, 79br Advertising Archives; 80l Rex Features/Steve Wood, 80b Natasha Pettigrew/Caroline Neville Associates; 81 Rex Features/Steve Wood; 81t Natasha Pettigrew/Caroline Neville Associates, 82b Rex Features; 83tl & ml Advertising Archives, 83tr, m, mr & bl Natasha Pettigrew/Caroline Neville Associates, 83br courtesy Ralph Lauren/Bruce Weber; 84t & bl courtesy Revlon; 85 all courtesy Revlon; 86tl, ml & b courtesy Revlon, 86tr Octavian/De Agostini UK, 86m IGDA; 87t, tr, mr & b courtesy Revlon, 87ml Advertising Archives; 88 all courtesy Shiseido; 89 all courtesy Shiseido; 90 all courtesy Shiseido; 91 all courtesy Shiseido except bl Octavian/De Agostini UK; 92l courtesy Balenciaga; 93 both courtesy Balenciaga; 94 all courtesy Balenciaga; 95 all courtesy Balenciaga; 96 both courtesy Rochas/ Variations PR; 97 both courtesy Rochas; 98t, bl & br Rochas; 98tr C. Di Pace; 99tl Farabolafoto, 99r, m & b courtesy Rochas; 100 courtesy Balmain; 101t courtesy Balmain, 101m Hulton Getty/Keystone; 102tl, tr, m & b courtesy Balmain, 102ml Advertising Archives; 103t, tr & ml courtesy Balmain, 103br Camera Press; 104 courtesy Cacharel; 105t courtesy Cacharel/Sarah Moon, 105b courtesy Parfums Beauté Italia; 106t & bl courtesy Cacharel/Jacques Dirand, 106br Advertising Archives; 107tl courtesy Cacharel, 107tr & br Cacharel, 107m & bl Parfums Beauté Italia, 107ml Advertising Archives, 107mr Green Moon Ltd.; 108t courtesy Floris, 108b IGDA, 109 both courtesy Floris; 110tl, bl & br courtesy Floris, 110tr & m IGDA; 111tr & b courtesy Floris, 111ml & mr Octavian/De Agostini UK; 112l & r courtesy Lanvin, 113l & r courtesy Lanvin; 114tr, tl & b courtesy Lanvin; 115tr, bl & r courtesy Lanvin, 115tl IGDA; 116t Farabolafoto, 116b courtesy Moschino, 117t & b courtesy Moschino, 117m Farabolafoto; 118t & m courtesy Moschino, 118b Farabolafoto; 119t & m courtesy Moschino, 119b Farabolafoto; 120 courtesy Avon; 121 courtesy Avon; 122 courtesy Avon; 123 courtesy Avon; 124 courtesy Patou/Balmain; 125t courtesy Patou/Balmain, 125b courtesy Caron; 126 courtesy Caron; 127tl & bl courtesy Caron; 127tr, ml & bm courtesy Patou/Balmain, 127mr Advertising Archives, 127br IGDA.